Rapid Research Methods for Nurses, Midwives and Health Professionals

Rapid Research Methods for Nurses, Midwives and Health Professionals

Colin Rees
Lecturer (retired)
School of Health Care Sciences
Cardiff University
Cardiff, UK

WILEY Blackwell

'For my wife Brenda, with thanks for her help and support'

Contents

Introduction, xi

Abstract, 1
Accidental sampling, 1
Action research, 2
Aim, 3
Analysis of Variance (ANOVA), 4
Analysis of Covariance (ANCOVA), 5
Anonymity, 6
Audit, 7
Audit trail, 8
Back chaining, 9
Bar graph, 10
Before and after designs, 11
Beneficence, 12
Bias, 13
Blinding, 14
Bracketing, 15
Case–control study, 16
Causal relationship, 17
Cell, 18
Chi-square test (χ^2), 19
Clinical trial, 19
Closed (close-ended, fixed choice) questions, 20
Cluster sample, 21
Coding, 22
Cohort study, 23
Concept definition, 24
Confidentiality, 25
Confirmability, 26
Confounding variable, 27
Contingency table, 27
Control group, 28
Convenience sample, 29
Correlation, 30
Covert observation, 31
Credibility, 32
Cross-over design, 33
Cross-sectional study, 34

Critique, 35
Data, 36
Database, 37
Data saturation, 38
Demographic data, 39
Dependent variable, 40
Descriptive statistics, 41
Double-blind study, 42
Ethics, 43
Ethics committee, 45
Ethnographic research, 46
Exclusion criteria, 46
Experimental design, 47
Ex post facto studies, 49
Face validity, 50
Fieldwork diary, 51
Fieldwork, 52
Findings, 53
Fittingness, 54
Focus group, 55
Forward chaining, 56
Frequency distribution, 57
Generalisability, 58
Grey literature, 59
Grounded theory, 60
Hawthorne effect, 61
Hermeneutics, 62
Heterogeneity and homogeneity, 63
Hierarchy of evidence, 64
Histogram, 65
Homogeneity, 65
Hypothesis, 66
Inclusion and exclusion criteria, 67
Inferential statistics, 68
Independent variable, 69
Informed consent, 70
Interval data, 70
Interviews, 71
Inverse relationship, 72
Judgemental sample, 73
Justice, 73
Key informant, 74
Key words, 75
Levels of measurement, 76

Likert scale, 78
Literature review, 79
Manipulation, 80
Masking, 80
Measures of central tendency, 81
Mean, 81
Measures of dispersion, 82
Meta-analysis, 83
Mode, 83
Median, 83
Naturalistic research, 84
Non-maleficence, 84
Nominal data, 84
Non-probability sampling methods, 85
Normal distribution, 86
Null hypothesis, 86
Observation, 87
Observational designs, 88
Open questions, 89
Operational definition, 90
Opportunity sample, 90
Outliers, 91
Ordinal data, 91
p Values, 92
Paradigm, 95
Phenomenology, 96
PICO, 96
Pilot study, 97
Population, 98
Power analysis, 99
Pretest–posttest designs, 99
Principles of research, 100
Probability sampling methods, 100
Prospective and retrospective study designs, 101
Qualitative research designs, 102
Quantitative research designs, 104
Quasi-experimental research, 105
Questionnaires, 106
Quota sampling, 106
Randomisation, 107
Randomised controlled trials (RCTs), 108
Range, 108
Ratio data, 108
Reflexivity, 108

Reliability, 109
Research, 110
Research design, 111
Research method, 112
Response rate, 112
Retrospective study, 112
Review of the literature, 112
Rigour, 113
Sample, 114
Sampling methods, 114
Sampling frame, 116
Self-report, 116
Snowball sample, 116
Social desirability, 116
Statistical analysis, 116
Survey, 117
Systematic reviews of the literature, 117
Table, 118
Thick data, 119
Transferability, 119
Triangulation, 119
Trustworthiness, 119
Type I, Type II, Type III errors, 120
Unstructured interviews, 122
Unstructured observations, 123
Validity, 124
Variable, 126

Introduction

The skill of understanding research reports and relating them to clinical practice is an essential part of being a health professional. However, understanding the language of research can be a considerable challenge as there are not only many unfamiliar words to learn, but those that are familiar, such as 'significant', have a different meaning from their everyday use. A useful solution to is an easy-to-read quick reference book that will explain key words as well as some of the 'need to know' principles on the topic.

This new addition to the 'Rapid' series takes some of the most frequently used words in research and reveals their meaning in simple terms and explains how they are applied in context. There are many of the same features as those already in the 'Rapid' series, including the use of helpful headings under each entry. The emphasis of the book is on helping healthcare students and qualified health professionals who already have some knowledge of research, to increase and consolidate their understanding of research.

In using this book, it is worth stressing that it is not an 'introduction to research', nor is it a stand-alone 'all you need to know about research' textbook. You will still need a comprehensive research textbook as well as some expert guidance. However, if you are just starting a research course or module, this book will be of great benefit, as it works as a helpful guide and useful rapid reference and revision book to accompany the more elaborate and complex textbooks.

Aim

The aim of this book is to increase your understanding of key research terminology and principles of research. It is different from the many available research textbooks as it uses easy to-understand language to link the meaning and ideas behind research concepts to some of the broader methodological principles. In this way, their relevance and implications can be better understood. The emphasis throughout is on explanation and understanding, so this is far more than just a glossary of research terms. The more you use it, the more you will see the bigger picture of research emerge.

If you are a student, you will find the book invaluable for developing critical analysis. It includes advice and tips for completing assignments, and its focus on the meaning of research terms will also be essential for multiple choice question (MCQ) papers. Its biggest advantage is that it helps the reader make connections between related entries and reveals some essential research ideas and principles. In other words, it enables you to build up your knowledge by applying the terminology to research processes and critical evaluation wherever in the book you start.

The structure

For speed and ease of access, the key research terms selected for this book are listed in alphabetical order. Each entry consists of the following headings:

Related to: This immediately places each word in context by listing other research terms with which it is generally associated.

Definition: A brief, clear and simply worded definition of the term.

Application: How the ideas behind the word are used in practice with an emphasis on the appropriate research or critiquing process.

Key revision points : A summary of the most important points that will get results when critically evaluating studies, writing research assignments or answering MCQs.

See also: This final heading provides the link to other closely related words in the book that should also be consulted.

Using this book

There is no correct way to use this book; it depends on how you want to use it and what works for you. As a suggestion, you can use this book alongside other research texts to speed up and consolidate the learning process. Use it when you come across a term or explanation that does not seem clear to you. This book will give you another point of view in understanding a concept. It may also give you a clearer understanding of the terminology or relevance of a research term.

If you are using this book for revision, then you have a number of options. You can make your own list of words that you feel require a more in-depth understanding. Once you have checked words here, you can return on a future occasion, cover the detail under the key word and see how much you remember.

An entertaining 'serendipity' way of using the book is to sit down, perhaps with a hot or cold drink, open the book anywhere and read through the next 10 words you find, or use the 'see also' suggestions to take you in different directions. Make notes on any key points that are revealed through your reading. This will quickly develop your research vocabulary and take you into words and ideas that you may not have discovered, or did not realise were connected.

Whichever method you use, you should find this book improves your fluency in research, almost without realising how much you are retaining. Its success will be apparent when you read research articles and find how much more sense they make! You should also find that when you are writing research assignments, critically evaluating articles or taking part in discussions on research, it suddenly becomes a lot easier and enjoyable subject. Research has a great potential to improve the quality of healthcare and this book has been designed to support you in playing your part in applying research to practice.

Colin Rees
Cardiff

Abstract

Related to: Research publications.

Definition: Overview of an article that briefly provides the main elements of a study.

Application: Used by a reader to consider the relevance of a study for a particular purpose or as a part of browsing an article to get an understanding of its content before either reading in detail or rejecting it.

Key revision points: Useful way of checking type of study, aim, results and recommendations of a study before reading through the full article itself. Look in particular at the aim, outcome measure, the intervention (if quantitative research) and conclusion to get a quick insight into the study. Consider how the study may contribute to your developing knowledge on its topic.

See also: Critique, aim, quantitative research.

Accidental sampling (See: Convenience sampling, sampling methods)

Rapid Research Methods for Nurses, Midwives and Health Professionals,
First Edition. Colin Rees.
© 2016 John Wiley & Sons, Ltd. Published 2016 by John Wiley & Sons, Ltd.

Action research

Related to: Research Design.

Definition: A research design involving the introduction of change and its evaluation. It is usually the result of collaboration between researchers and practitioners. Such studies consist of the design and analysis of service change followed by the repetition of these steps until a suitable solution or improvement has been achieved.

Application: It provides a quick method to change the delivery of services in a controlled and evaluated way. Although many examples are available, it is still not a commonly used within healthcare.

Key revision points: This method differs from the usual researcher-led design in healthcare. It requires close agreement and working harmony between the researchers and practitioners to identify the nature of a service or organisational problem and its possible solution. Both parties must then work together on its implementation and evaluation. The advantage of action research is its immediacy, as planned change is introduced not as a recommendation but as the focus of the study. There are usually a number of stages to such studies where the cycle of plan–implement–evaluate–repeat leads to slight changes or adjustments until it is agreed that a successful solution to the original problem has been reached. The method of evaluation will use carefully designed research methods (tools) and analysis.

There are some arguments about whether action research is a true research method as there are limitations on the extent to which knowledge gained in such a study can be generalised. However, examples of its beneficial use can be found in the nursing and midwifery literature.

See also: Research design.

Aim (also called objective or purpose)

Related to: The research process, the research question.

Definition: A statement of the purpose of the study that gives the study design direction, as data are collected to answer the aim.

Application: The researcher develops the aim at the start of the planning process. In research articles, it can be found in the abstract and in the main body, usually at the end of the literature review or introduction, and immediately before the section 'methods'. It often starts with the words 'the aim of this study was to determine/examine/explore, etc.'.

Key revision points: Once the aim of a study is written, it will shape other aspects of the design as the wording and content will make many of the stages of a study follow prescribed ways to answer the question to be answered. For example, aims that set out to compare outcomes will usually take the form of a randomised controlled trial (RCT); aims that seek to explore something are generally qualitative studies. In experimental designs, there can be a hypothesis related to the aim that the research sets out to test (the word 'prove' is not used as this is very difficult to establish). When critiquing a study, locate the aim then jump to the conclusion to check if the researcher has clearly answered it. The conclusion should include wordings similar to the aim; if it does not, you may not have found the true conclusion.

See also: Hypothesis, Type III Error.

Analysis of Variance (ANOVA)

Related to: Experimental designs, randomised control trials, hypotheses, statistical analysis.

Definition: In experimental research, a statistical method of testing a hypothesis to assess the existence of a difference between three or more groups in relation to a specific outcome measure (dependent variable). The mean (average) scores or measures between groups are used in the calculation. ANOVA can also be used in non-experimental studies, such as surveys, to test the effect of a number of variables on an outcome measure.

Application: In clinical RCTs, participants can be allocated to three or more groups, each one receiving a different intervention. ANOVA is used to measure the differences found in the groups in relation to the outcome measure so that the more successful interventions can be identified. In descriptive studies, the researcher is sometimes interested in the influence of a number of factors or measures that are not introduced by a researcher but part of the experience or characteristic of those in the sample that can be clustered into groups and its influence on an outcome measured. Characteristics can include age group, or gender, length of treatment or intensity or strength of treatment and an outcome measure such as level of reported pain, hours of sleep per night, or level of anxiety. ANOVA will identify which variables seem to be linked to the outcome measure.

Key revision points: 'ANOVA' is created by combining letters from the phrase **AN**alysis **O**f **VA**riance. It demonstrates the rigour of the researcher in applying statistical processes to compare the means (average results) between groups in an experimental study and a number of variations that might influence any differences discovered between them. It has a long and popular history and is highly regarded as a way of establishing whether a hypothesis should be accepted or rejected, or in non-experimental studies, to identify which factors or attributes appear to have an effect on outcomes. In assignment work, it may be sufficient to recognise the use of this technique as a clear indication that it is a well-conducted study where the data have been processed correctly and the researchers have supported their conclusions.

See also: Analysis of covariance, hypotheses, randomised control trials, inferential statistics.

Analysis of Covariance (ANCOVA)

Related to: Experimental designs, especially randomised control trials, hypotheses, statistical analysis.

Definition: Statistical tests used in a similar way to ANOVA (see the previous entry) but take into account the effect of one or more variables not controlled in an RCT design that may affect outcome measures between groups.

Application: Goes one step further than the ANOVA, by taking account of factors outside the control of the researcher that might influence the results, which is why it is called the 'analysis of covariance'.

Key revision points: It is similarly an indicator of the rigour of the researcher in searching for statistical relationships in the data that will help to explain the results in an experimental design study.

See also: ANOVA, hypotheses, randomised control trials, inferential statistics.

Anonymity

Related to: Research ethics.

Definition: The protection of the identity of an individual or setting in a study by not revealing a name, characteristic, location or any other feature that would provide clues as to the source of the data and the individual people involved.

Application: Researchers are under an ethical obligation to design and carry out their work so that it is not possible to identify individuals or locations involved in data collection. This is part of the attempt to do no harm (non-maleficence) to those in a study. Individuals could be put at a disadvantage if personal details about them were known to others. This is the same issue as that related to confidentiality in clinical practice.

Key revision points: Researchers should indicate that they have followed the principle of anonymity in published work. Health premises used as the site for studies should be given a general description such as 'a large city hospital', 'the local clinical area' to prevent an educated guess as to participants. Individuals may be given a number, for example, 'Respondent 1 or (R1)', or a pseudonym, for example, 'Molly'. Protecting the identity of individuals is a key aspect in ethical rigour of studies. It may also help individuals to feel that they can be more honest and open in providing information in a study and so increase the level of validity in the study.

See also: Ethics, rigour.

Audit

Definition: The systematic collection of clinical or performance data to compare with standards, targets or baseline measures.

Application: Audit is commonly used in many clinical and organisational settings to monitor the quality of care against targets or standards. The methods it uses to collect data include the use of records, questionnaires, interviews and observation.

Key revision points: Audit is not regarded as a research activity, although it frequently looks like it, and is sometimes presented as if it were research. However, although the findings may be interesting, it only produces information relevant to the location in which it was carried out; it does not produce transferable knowledge about a topic in the same way that research adds to our general knowledge and understanding. Nevertheless, it should be carried out with the same rigour as research using a reasonable sample size and reliable tools of data collection. Emphasise your knowledge that there is a difference between audit and research when referring to it in written work or conversation.

See also: Generalisability, research, principles of research.

Audit trail

Related to: Qualitative research, data analysis.

Definition: In the presentation of qualitative research study, the inclusion of details on the method of analysis that allows a reader to trace how the researcher went from in-depth interviews to the theme headings used to present the data. This provides transparency in the process followed.

Application: In the 'methods' section of published research, and often also in the findings, the qualitative researcher should make it clear how they followed a standardised and systematic process in analysing the volume of verbal, observational or written material they have gathered. The audit trail is the visible path outlined by the researcher showing how they have clustered and condensed the data into meaningful 'units of text' and eventually theme headings. Authors can describe the process in the text, or it may be shown visually in boxes or figures.

Key revision points: This is different from the concept of audit included in the previous entry. Here, the audit trail is a key aspect to include when critiquing qualitative research. Its presence is a way of reassuring the reader that analytical rigour has been applied in the study. Just as in financial auditing, in qualitative research, the author must be persuasive and transparent in the way in which they have processed and analysed their data if the findings are to be trusted.

See also: Qualitative research.

Back chaining

Related to: Searching the literature.

Definition: When reviewing the literature, this is the use of the reference lists in articles as a way of finding further relevant publications.

Application: A review of the literature is produced following a comprehensive search of the literature for as much relevant material as possible. In addition to the use of keywords and databases to find articles, a useful search method is to examine the reference list at the end of good quality and recent articles you have already found.

Key revision points: Back chaining is a way of gaining relevant articles that may have been missed in a database search. An important disadvantage of this method is that the 'chain' will take you further back into the past into quite 'old' literature. For this reason, use more recent articles first when using this method or use 'forward chaining'.

See also: Literature review, forward chaining, key words.

Rapid Research Methods for Nurses, Midwives and Health Professionals,
First Edition. Colin Rees.
© 2016 John Wiley & Sons, Ltd. Published 2016 by John Wiley & Sons, Ltd.

Bar graph

Related to: Data analysis, data presentation.

Definition: A visual method of displaying numeric data in the form of blocks.

Application: Visual display techniques such as bar graphs provide an easy way to compare different groups or results in a study. Bar charts can be shown vertically, extending up the page, or horizontally, extending across the page.

Key revision points: Although they look similar, bar graphs are different from their near neighbour, the histogram. Bar graphs show one variable measured in terms of 'nominal' (or categorical) data (number within one group or another). These include data not expressed in a numerical measurement (e.g. age), and can only be counted in terms of frequency, for example, the number of males or females, the number in each category of causes of falls in elderly hospital patients. Each bar in a bar graph displays the number of items or number of times each category was counted and is indicated by the height of the bar.

Histograms collect a different type of data: those that can be broken down and measured along a continuum, for example, height, age, weight. For this reason, the bars in a bar graph do not touch, but those in a histogram do as they are measured along a continuum at the bottom of the graph. Care has to be taken with bar graphs as the differences between each bar can be exaggerated by using a large scale. This would show a big difference in the height of each bar that in reality may only be a small number. When interpreting bar charts, take into account the scale used to present them.

Both bar groups and histograms have the figure number and title below the figure as figures are usually read from the bottom up. In contrast, tables are numbered and titled above the table as tables are read down (see Figure 1).

See also: Histograms.

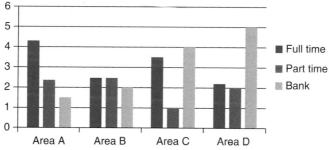

Figure 1 Bar chart showing number of staff in each category of employment in four clinical areas.

Before and after designs (pretest–posttest designs)

Related to: Research designs, experimental designs.

Definition: A form of experimental design where subjects (individuals, events or objects) are firstly measured in relation to the outcome measure(s) before any intervention (the 'before' or 'pre' stage), and then measured again following the intervention (the 'after' or 'post' stage) in order to see if those in the experimental group improve compared with the control group.

Application: A randomised controlled trial is the strongest form of research for demonstrating that an intervention is successful. Although they can take many forms, the classic design is to randomly allocate a group of consenting subjects to an experimental and control group, and measure the dependent variable (outcome measure) at the start of the study, apply an intervention and control, and re-measure at least once after the intervention. The study requires a great deal of skill in its execution and analysis; the reward is the ability to produce convincing results of a cause-and-effect relationship that will be relevant to practice or to increasing knowledge.

Key revision points: The 'before–after' design (also known as pretest–posttest design) is where the two groups are measured at two or more points in time in order to build up the evidence of a cause-and-effect relationship. This design has considerable credibility when carried out to a high standard, as it makes any other explanation other than the experimental intervention unlikely. However, it is important to check that the groups are equally matched at the beginning (the variables that might affect the outcome should show a non-significant or 'NS' statistical difference between the two groups at the beginning). Once the intervention has been introduced, the 'after' measurements should show that the dependent variable (outcome measure) in the experimental group is statistically different from the control group following the intervention.

See also: Experimental design.

Beneficence

Related to: Ethical principles.

Definition: The basic ethical principle of doing good through an intervention or action. Research must have at least the potential of producing a beneficial effect if it is to be approved. The actions of the researcher must promote and not endanger this principle.

Application: Where a study involves individuals or is conducted in health settings, an ethics committee must consider if it will improve knowledge or care. It should also be clear in the research proposal that the way the study is to be conducted will promote and protect the human rights of those taking part.

Key revision points: Beneficence is often talked about at the same time as non-maleficence. These two terms basically mean similar things: the first relates to actions that result in 'doing good' and the second to actions that result in 'avoiding harm'. In assignment and exam work, demonstrate your knowledge of this technical language through the use of terms such as 'beneficence' and illustrate your understanding by explaining its meaning.

See also: Ethics.

Bias

Related to: The research process, sampling.

Definition: Any aspect of a study that distorts or skews the results or interpretation of the results.

Application: In designing a study, the researcher should consider if there is anything that may negatively influence the accuracy of the results and try to reduce these as much as possible. For example, the researcher should try to ensure that those in a quantitative study represent a good cross-section of those found in the larger population the study examines. Too many of those in an unrepresentative subgroup will lead to a distortion in the data and skew the conclusions drawn. Examples would include an imbalance of males or females in a study that did not reflect the proportions normally found in a setting. In randomised controlled trials, bias can also emerge as a result of subjects, staff or data collectors knowing if individuals are in the experimental or control group. For this reason, a number of precautions are taken to ensure that it is not clear who is in which group. This takes the form of 'blinding', also called 'masking' of one or more parties involved (subjects/staff/data gathers), so that it is not known who is in which group. This will reduce conscious or unconscious distortion of the results.

Key revision points: The concept of bias is one of the key aspects of critically evaluating studies in the process of critiquing research articles. If bias has occurred, it can lead the researcher to incorrect conclusions, and so reduce the value of the study. Although some bias may be outside the control of researchers, they should still try and anticipate at what points a study may be vulnerable to bias and try to reduce it. When critiquing research, look particularly at the sample in a study and consider whether they are 'typical' of the larger group they represent. The first part of the results section in an article usually summarises the main characteristics of the study sample and is included for the purpose of allowing the reader to check the composition of the group. In randomised controlled studies, examine if blinding was possible and has taken place. Finally, consider if the researcher has taken possible bias into account in their 'limitations' of the study.

See also: Rigour, blinding, double-blind study, critique, experimental design.

Blinding

Related to: Experimental designs, randomised controlled trials.

Definition: The withholding or concealing of information on who has been allocated to the experimental or control group in a randomised controlled trial in order to reduce bias. Its purpose is to increase the accuracy of the results of a study.

Application: Randomised controlled trials are highly valued because of the care taken to limit the influence of factors that can distort or bias the results. Blinding is the attempt to ensure that participants and those providing care, or treatments, or those analysing results, do not know who is allocated to which group. This is because such knowledge may influence the behaviour of those in a study, and the assessments or interpretations of those involved in handling data.

Key revision points: Blinding is also known as 'masking' or 'concealment'. It should be discussed when critiquing randomised controlled trials in which blinding is possible.

It can take two forms: firstly, only withholding or hiding information on who was in which group from those in the study, or only those conducting the study or interpreting the results (single-blind) or secondly, concealing information from respondents as well as those carrying out the study or interpreting the results (double blind).

Particularly in medical research, this criterion has a high value, but in nursing research it is not always possible for masking to take place. This is because in nursing research the interventions in the experimental and control group are very different in appearance, and it is not possible to make them look similar or disguise their appearance, as is the case in medical research with the use of drugs. A clear example would be a midwifery study comparing the outcome of birthing in water compared with birthing in a bed; water cannot be disguised to look like a bed. Despite this, it is important where it is possible to conceal the type of intervention and for the researcher to do everything they can to minimise knowledge of the allocated group.

See also: Experimental designs, bias.

Bracketing

Related to: Qualitative research, phenomenology.

Definition: A technique applied by some phenomenological qualitative researchers to avoid contaminating the findings of a study. It is achieved by setting to one side or 'bracketing' the researcher's beliefs, opinions and experiences that might shape lines of enquiry with respondents or interpretation of the findings.

Application: In some phenomenological studies, as part of the attempt to demonstrate rigour, the researcher makes a conscious effort to consider their own views, experiences and preconceptions on the nature of the topic they are exploring. These are then 'bracketed' or put to one side, so that the respondent guides the interview agenda and so are not influenced by the researcher's personal expectations or past experiences.

Key revision points: This is a controversial area of phenomenological research that arose at the beginning of the twentieth century when the German philosopher Husserl proposed the need to set aside one's own experiences in order to examine ideas in a more objective way. By the 1920s, one of his students, Heidegger, had taken over Husserl's position as professor in Freiberg University, Germany, and held very different views on bracketing. He suggested that we cannot help but use our past experience in interpreting our world and suggested that it is not possible or desirable to bracket the experiences that shape us as individuals. In assignment work, rather than take sides on this argument, it is better to acknowledge that these contrasting views exist, and use this to understand the different forms taken by phenomenological research.

See also: Qualitative research, phenomenology.

Case–control study

Related to: Observational non-randomised research design.

Definition: A technique of comparing individuals with a condition (the cases) with those without the same condition, but similar in most other respects (the controls) by retro-spectively producing 'matched' pairs of people. This allows a researcher to observe what differences exist between the two groups that might have influenced the condition or outcome.

Application: It is not always possible, or desirable, to carry out a prospective randomised controlled trial (RCT) and allocate people to experimental and control groups where some form of manipulation of their treatment takes place. One alternative is to look back through things such as records, self-reports or interviews and match people with and without a specific condition and to compare the details about them. The purpose is to estimate the influences of factors that might have influenced the condition and its progression.

Key revision points: This kind of study is categorised as an 'observational design' as the researcher does not introduce an intervention or independent variable, but observes the result of a natural exposure to a variable by those in the experimental group. It is associated with epidemiological research designs concerned with identifying factors that influence the development of clinical conditions. Unusually, it starts from a known clinical outcome that is different between the two groups and works back towards identifying which factors may have intervened and been influential in the development of the outcome. This idea differs from most experiments in many ways, for example, the researcher does not introduce anything (a major feature of experiments) and unlike experiments it is *retrospective* (the data already exist in the past) rather than *prospective* (the outcome is unknown as the data lie in the future).

When critiquing such studies, the researcher's inclusion and exclusion criteria for the sample should be carefully examined to ensure that the two groups are as similar as possible; only the presence of the condition or attribute being studied should be the major difference between them.

As a case–control study is retrospective in design, it comes under the heading of an '*ex post facto*' study, that is, it looks at a situation 'after the fact' of developing a condition. There are many limitations to such studies related to the design, for example, the diffi-culty of gathering subjects who are a reasonable 'match'. The availability and accuracy of retrospective data can also be a problem. In addition, such studies cannot identify cause-and-effect relationships but only associations (correlation). The common statistics used in these studies is the odds ratio (OR), which establishes the odds that the two groups are different in relation to specific factors.

See also: Observational designs, ex post facto studies, prospective studies.

Rapid Research Methods for Nurses, Midwives and Health Professionals,
First Edition. Colin Rees.
© 2016 John Wiley & Sons, Ltd. Published 2016 by John Wiley & Sons, Ltd.

Causal relationship

Related to: Experimental designs, statistical analysis.

Definition: The existence of a statistically demonstrated relationship between two variables where one (the independent variable) can be seen to have a direct and predictable effect (outcome) on the other (the dependent variable).

Application: Experimental designs, such as RCTs, are designed to test for causality, which can be demonstrated statistically by processing the results using a test of significance. This calculates the extent to which such a relationship has been demonstrated in the study. Causality can be confirmed providing there is a clear and strong relationship demonstrated by the test of statistical significance.

The independent variable (the intervention) must have been introduced before measuring its possible impact on the outcome measure (the dependent variable), and the observed outcome should always occur whenever the independent variable is introduced. As there are so many influences on a study's outcomes, researchers avoid stating they have 'proved' the existence of a relationship, preferring to make more cautious statements such as 'it has been demonstrated' or 'suggested' by the results.

Key revision points: The search for causal relationships is a frequent driver for healthcare research. The usual research design chosen to demonstrate a causal relationship is that of the randomised controlled trail (RCT). This is because of the control the researcher has over other explanations of the outcome other than the experimental intervention. Other relationships, such as correlation, are possible in studies but these do not demonstrate a causal relationship.

See also: Hypothesis, 'p' values, experimental design, correlation.

Cell

Related to: Presentation of results, data analysis.

Definition: One segment or square of a table showing the numeric results of a study. It contains one value, which can be displayed as a raw number and/or percentage, and occurs at the point at which a column and row meet.

Application: Part of the researcher's role is to provide the reader with meaningful data. The presentation of the data in tables is a familiar method of grouping the results and identifying possible patterns in the variables under study. The results of a study must be clear and allow the reader to search for patterns themselves, or clearly notice those described by the author.

Key revision points: When faced with tables look carefully at the title of the table as this will describe the picture the table presents, then look at the headings used in the columns and rows so that you can be clear on what a particular cells represent, for example, result of the number of women with 'severe' pain. Check if the number in a cell is the raw (actual) number, or a percentage, or if it contains both. Percentages alone can be misleading unless you establish the actual number they represent. This avoids mistaking a large percentage in a cell as representing a large number of people; for example, a finding that 66.6% of people had not seen their GP in over a year in a sample of three people represents two responses! There are no restrictions on the number of cells per table, but the larger the table the more difficult it can be to interpret and the more intimidating it can look. A frequently used format is the 2 by 2 (2×2) table, which has two rows and two columns and is a form of cross-tabulation.

See also: Critiquing, statistics.

Chi-square test (χ^2)

Related to: Statistics, quantitative analysis, relationships between variables.

Definition: A common statistical test to examine relationships between attributes or variables in quantitative research that take a 'nominal' (naming) form, that is, they are either in one discrete category or another with no in-between points as with age or temperature, for example, male/female, yes/no.

Application: In surveys and some experimental methods, the frequency of variables or characteristics of a sample are collected and shown in a table to establish if a pattern can be identified between those involved and the variables examined. A chi-square test is used to establish if the frequencies (the number in each category) are the same as, or different from, the frequencies that could have been expected or anticipated if there was no real difference between the groups examined.

For example, in a survey on nutrition are females more likely to eat five fruits/vegetables per day compared with males? The categories are male/female and yes/no in relation to eating a minimum of five fruits/vegetables per day. The test compares the number of females answering 'yes' with the number of males answering 'yes' and calculates if there is a difference greater than if there had been no difference between the groups. This calculation tests what is called 'the null hypothesis', that is, the hypothesis that both groups are the same – no difference between them. A greater-than-expected result would suggest that the two groups are different and a pattern does exist between the groups and the variable examined. This may help in planning healthcare interventions.

Key revision points: The name of the test is pronounced 'ki' to rhyme with 'try'. UK books tend to refer to the 'chi-square' test and US books refer to the 'chi-squared' test; both spellings are acceptable.

This statistical test can only be used with 'nominal' data. This is also called categorical data, which makes the meaning of the term easier to understand; it is either in one category or another.

The test does not suggest a cause-and-effect relationship but is a measure of correlation, that is, there may be relationship in the form of a pattern of association. It is a popular and frequently used test and requires the use of the actual number in each group examined rather than the percentage.

See also: Statistics, levels of measurements.

Clinical trial (See: Randomised controlled trial)

Closed (close-ended, fixed choice) questions

Related to: Questionnaires and interviews.

Definition: A method of asking questions in either questionnaires or interviews where the respondent can only choose from a small number of options offered.

Application: A number of research studies collect data by asking respondents questions, where their answer is chosen from a list of given options such as 'Would you say your health is (a) better than yesterday or (b) about the same as yesterday or (c) worse than yesterday or (d) undecided?'
These are closed questions as the freedom to answer in one's own words is 'closed' to the individual.

Key revision points: This type of questions makes analysis a lot easier as the frequency that each option is chosen is counted and easily shown in tables It is a simple operation for computer-based analysis. The disadvantage is that the choices offered may not reflect how the respondent really feels, and this can affect the accuracy of the results (validity). This type of question is also called 'fixed-choice' and 'cafeteria question', both of which highlight the 'choosing from a list' approach to answering. The opposite of a closed question is an open question, for example, 'Can you tell me how you are feeling today compared to yesterday?'

See also: Open questions, questionnaires, survey.

Cluster sample

Related to: Sampling methods.

Definition: A method of selecting the sample in the form of groups or 'clusters' of units rather than individuals. This is part of multiple-stage sampling where the researcher starts with broad units, such as geographical areas, and gradually through choosing structures at increasingly lower levels, such as hospitals, then clinical units and ends by including all those in predetermined level of selection, for example, ward or clinical area.

Application: In large surveys, it can be difficult to ensure that a representative broad sample is selected from the target population and data collected from them at a reasonable cost and effort. Although the random sample method is the ideal choice, it requires a complete list or sampling frame of all those eligible from which the sample is selected, and the sample may be very thinly spread over a large geographical area. The alternative is to step down in size order from randomly selected larger locations, such as counties, then hospitals, then clinical areas from appropriate sampling frames and finally include everyone in the smaller areas identified. This gives rise to the alternative name for this system, which is multi-stage sampling.

Key revision points: Sampling methods vary in the extent to which they produce a group of respondents whose results can be generalised to a wide population. Probability sampling methods are those that produce more accurate results; cluster sampling is one of the methods in this category and can be quicker, cheaper and as accurate as the alternative of the random sample. It is accomplished through the use of phases of diminishing sized levels, allowing the use of accessible sampling frames and then including all those who 'cluster' in the final level. The advantage is that instead of being spread out and expensive to cover, the sample is concentrated in a smaller area and therefore easier to access. However, there are a number of disadvantages; for example, the resulting group of individuals can be quite small, and if taken from just one area/unit may have characteristics not necessarily shared with other excluded areas, both of these limitations may produce a greater level of sampling error (inaccurate results) but this can be outweighed by the system's advantages.

See also: Sampling methods.

Coding

Related to: Qualitative research, analysis.

Definition: A method of data analysis in qualitative research where the large amount of text gathered through interviews and/or observation is broken down into smaller headings or description. Each of these separate units of meaning is allocated a category label or 'code' by the researcher. These can be clustered under more general headings to identify emerging themes that describe the findings.

Application: Coding is a stepping stone to the final analysis process that allows the researcher to build up an understanding of what is going on in a qualitative study. It requires the researcher to carefully, and often repeatedly, read through each line of the findings and consider a heading or title that could be used as a 'file heading' under which a sentence or large piece of description/dialogue could be placed, for example, 'building a defence against failure', or 'knowing one's limits'. In grounded theory, the coding process is often carried out in three hierarchical stages:

   i) Level one: open coding, where each sentence or 'unit of text' is given a code

   ii) Level two: coding – the bringing together of related codes into clusters

   iii) Level three: 'axial' coding – developing wider theme headings under which clusters can be grouped or ordered.

There are other forms of coding used in a variety of qualitative approaches all consisting of a process of reading and re-reading the findings, and applying increasingly focussed levels of codes to the data.

Key revision points: Coding is a good example of a systematic way in which qualitative research is carried out. It also illustrates rigour in qualitative research. Coding is a difficult process, and its accuracy is more convincing when illustrated with examples of content covered by codes, clusters and themes. When critiquing, look out for examples of these illustrations in the form of extracts from raw data. Sometimes, articles will provide an 'audit trial' to show examples of open coding that have been grouped together into clusters and finally given an overall theme heading.

Although usually associated with qualitative research, coding can be used in quantitative surveys to analyse open comments in some questions. This would still make the study quantitative but containing some qualitative data to add a little more depth or understanding to the numeric findings.

See also: Audit trail, data analysis, rigour.

Cohort study

Related to: Research design, observational studies.

Definition: A longitudinal observational research design that studies a group of people who share an experience, characteristic or condition in common over time. The purpose is to establish the risk factors or exposure to developing conditions or reaction to treatment.

Application: Used in medical and epidemiological research to identify those with a condition of interest and the effect of exposure to variables that are either naturally occurring or selected by individuals. This is in contrast to RCTs where the researcher deliberately introduces a treatment or intervention in a controlled situation. In a cohort study, the researcher observes the effect of factors on the course of the individual's health or recovery that would not be possible in an RCT due to ethical problems such as deliberately introducing or withholding exposure to an intervention. It can also be a cheaper method of study.

Key revision points: This is a useful approach to gathering knowledge about specific groups sharing a specific age, for example, children or the older person, or a condition, such as diabetes or cancer. It is less ethically sensitive in design as the researcher simply observes and records progress over time and does not interfere with prescribed or self-selected treatments or activity. The design is described as longitudinal and can be prospective, that is, collects data into the future, or retrospective, that is, collects data that has already happened or been created.
An alternative to a longitudinal study would be a cross-sectional study that would look at one group at one point in time but at different stages of the variable under examination, or different points in their experience, for example, nursing students in different years of study, but collected at the same time. A cohort study is not as strong a design as an RCT as it lacks the control by the researcher to limit the influence of other factors that might affect outcomes. In addition, there is not a control element to provide comparative data. The representativeness of the individuals can be an issue. Similarly, the number of people who are forced to drop out, or decide to leave the study (referred to as study 'mortality' although the reason may not be death), can also weaken the strength of the results.

See also: Longitudinal studies, prospective studies, RCTs.

Concept definition

Related to: Variables, critiquing, data analysis.

Definition: The meaning of a key word, concept or variable in a study that provides the definition or meaning of the word as used in the study.

Application: Many words can be open to several meanings, particularly abstract terms such as 'resistance' or 'quality of life'. In research, it is important that where a variable is to be measured, the researcher is clear on what exactly they are looking for and to only include examples of that variable, otherwise it calls into question the validity of the data. Researchers will examine available alternative meanings of the term and will either chose an existing definition or create their own. This should be stated in the study so that everyone reading the study will have a common understanding of what the term means within the context of the study. For example, 'Pain has been defined in this study as an unpleasant feeling of discomfort or distress that results in physical or emotional negative sensations'.

Key revision points: The existence of concept definitions for the main variables in a study is important for both those carrying out a study and those reading it to ensure that a common language exists between both parties. As part of critical analysis, identify concept definitions and consider their clarity: do you feel it provides a description that would prevent misunderstandings? If you were given the definition and told to find examples of it, for example, patients with emotional resilience, could you correctly identify them? It can be problematic if the researcher has not thought to provide concept definitions for key variables as they can become vague or ambiguous.

Concept definitions are also crucial when reviewing the literature to ensure that different studies can be compared or combined. Unless authors in different studies have used similar concept definitions, it will be difficult to compare them, as you may not be comparing like with like. This could make a world of difference to how the findings are combined or used in practice. It is also important to know how concepts are measured within studies for the same reason; this is referred to as an *operational definition*, for example, an operational definition of pain could be a pain scale measuring degree of perceived pain from 0 to 10, where 10 is the highest level of pain.

See also: Operational definition, validity, variable.

Confidentiality

Related to: Ethics.

Definition: Ensuring that sensitive or private information is not included in a research report or made public. This extends to any information that would reveal or make it easy to guess the identity of an individual or location.

Application: Part of the ethical principles of research include anonymity, which is keeping an individual's identity hidden, and confidentiality, which is not sharing information that may harm an individual or be undesirable for others to discover. The role of the researcher is to guard against breaches in confidentiality by ensuring that the study has been approved by a relevant ethical review body, and that all those taking part in a study have provided informed consent to participate. In addition, any research data must be stored so that they cannot be accessed by those not involved in the study and that it is disposed of in line with the guidance given for the study.

Key revision points: Although the technical aspects of a study are crucial to the quality of the findings, ethical standards are even more important. Ethical rigour is one of the key elements in any study as it demonstrates that the work is ethically sound; without it most journals will refuse to publish the work. Despite this, in many current research articles, the depth of information on ethics can be very brief. However, providing a study has been agreed by an ethics committee it is unlikely that there should be any problems with ethical issues such as confidentiality. If names are used in relation to patients, which can be the case in qualitative research, the researcher will usually explain that these are pseudonyms, that is, they are not the real names of those involved.

See also: Ethics, informed consent, anonymity.

Confirmability

Related to: Assessing qualitative studies.

Definition: In qualitative research, the extent to which the findings can be judged as accurate and based on the data collected, and not simply the subjective views or interpretation of the researcher.

Application: The differences between quantitative and qualitative study designs mean that issues such as objectivity are difficult to compare. Here, the qualitative researcher must demonstrate an absence of their own bias or personal interpretation by illustrating how the analysis and interpretations can be backed up by the data in the study and therefore support the accuracy of the data.

Key revision points: In assignment work, it is expected that you will demonstrate familiarity with the different criteria for judging a qualitative study compared with a quantitative study. Reference to criteria developed by Lincoln and Guba (other references include Guba on his own, as well as Guba and Lincoln, which all cover similar points) are often seen in the literature. These involve criteria such as credibility, transferability, dependability and confirmability. These are not easy to understand as they are very close in meaning. Other terms such as fittingness and audit trail are also used. It is worth persevering with these terms to ensure a clear understanding of the major principles. They are all an attempt to establish how far we can have confidence in the accuracy of the study's findings and the interpretations offered by the author.

Confirmability is illustrated by the researcher's attempts to check that the study's findings can be supported by things such as a 'member's check', where those who provided data confirm the accuracy of the details having been shown transcripts of interviews or interpretations.

In a published study, the categories or headings used to present the findings should also be supported with examples of observations or dialogues that illustrate the terms developed. In qualitative studies, the use of more than one data collection method (triangulation) is also popular and used to support the accuracy of the findings. Where the elements of credibility, transferability and dependability are present in a study, it can be argued that confirmability has been established as it is an overriding or umbrella term.

See also: Credibility, transferability, dependability, fittingness, audit trail.

Confounding variable

Related to: *Statistics, analysis*

Definition: Those variables in a study that cannot be controlled by the researcher but can influence the outcome. These may or may not be recognised by the researcher.

Application: A great deal of quantitative research focusses on the search for relationships between variables. Researchers try to take account of variables that are outside the study design but that may influence the outcome; however, often their influence is not revealed until the study is in progress or has concluded. In the discussion section of the study, there may be a heading 'Limitations' where the researcher will comment on these confounding variables that may have influenced the results.

Key revision points: In critiquing studies, it is important to consider if the researcher had control over all the variables that may have played a part in the outcome of a study. Were there other confounding variables that might have had a strong influence on the outcome that has not been taken into account or fully acknowledged? This is particularly important in RCTs.

See also: Variables, critiquing.

Contingency table (See: Table)

Control group

Related to: Experimental design

Definition: The control group in an experimental design is the one that does not receive the intervention, that is, the experimental variable. Those in a control group are used as a comparison measure to establish what might have happened if those in the experimental group had not received the intervention under study.

Application: Experimental designs look for cause-and-effect relationships between an independent variable (an intervention) and a dependent variable (an outcome measure). The existence of such a relationship is strengthened by the use of a control group that is similar in all ways to the experimental group apart from one – exposure to the experimental variable. If the groups are alike in all ways apart from this one difference, then variations in the outcome can only be due to what is different between them – the experimental variable.

Control groups allow the researcher to say 'this is what would have happened if we had not introduced what we did'. It is hoped that there will be a difference between the two groups at the end of the experiment with regard to the outcome measure (dependent variable) and that the experimental group will show greater improvements than the control group, thus demonstrating that the experimental variable (the intervention) is more effective than whatever the control group experienced, usually either current practice or nothing, in the form of a placebo.

Key revision points: Those in a study must have an equal chance of being allocated to either the experimental or control group. If they are randomly allocated then not only have they had an equal chance of being allocated to either group, but there will also be an equal distribution of other factors that might have made a difference to the results. It is this match between experimental and control group that is crucial to the success of experimental designs. Some studies do not follow this format, having instead only one group that has both the experimental and alternative interventions. This is called a 'crossover' or 'within-subject' design, where individuals act as their own control.

See also: Experimental design, experimental group.

Convenience sample (also called an accidental or opportunity sample)

Related to: Sampling.

Definition: In sampling, those individuals who happen to be in the right place at the right time and who agree to be included in data gathering.

Application: Where the researcher does not have to be very precise in who is included in a study, this very practical or pragmatic method of selection is used. The alternative expressions for a convenience sample are 'accidental' and 'opportunity' sample and are well-chosen terms as they indicate how those in this kind of sample are recruited into a study – they just happen to be easily accessed. This includes stopping people in the street or in a health location and asking them if they are willing to take part.

Key revision points: This method of gaining respondents in a study comes under the heading of 'non-probability' sampling methods, and is ideal for exploring a new topic where the quality of representativeness of those in the sample is not a major concern. With this method, it is difficult to estimate how representative individuals are, due to the lack of control over who is included. As a consequence, the results may not be generalisable to the larger group. That is not to say the results are wrong, only that we have no way of telling how accurate they are. Despite the limitations, this is still a very popular way of selecting the sample.

See also: Sampling methods, probability and non-probability sampling methods

Correlation

Related to: Statistics, research designs.

Definition: A statistical relationship between variables that suggests the existence of a pattern or association between them. This is not the same as a causal relationship; instead, it suggests that the variables are related in some way demonstrated by variations in their measurements that are linked or patterned.

Application: A major aspect of quantitative research is the search for relationships between variables. This permits predictions to be made about interventions and likely outcomes, or the relationship between various patients or client attributes and environmental factors. The two main forms that these relationships take are cause-and-effect relationships, as in an RCT, and a correlation, or pattern in the relationships between two variables. A correlation identifies a link between values of one variable in relation to values in another, such as level of fitness and level of blood pressure. It is detected through the use of a calculation called a correlation coefficient that will indicate the strength (low/medium/high) and direction (positive or negative) of the correlation between the variables.

Key revision points: The two main correlation coefficients used in statistical calculations are *Pearson's Product Moment Correlation Coefficient (known as Pearson's 'r')* and *Spearman's Rank Order Correlation Coefficient (or Spearman's 'rho', pronounced 'row')*. The most important revision point is that a correlation does not indicate a 'cause-and-effect' relationship but an association relationship. There could be a third unknown variable that is influencing both variables and producing the pattern identified. A perfect correlation (e.g. where a rise of 10% in the value of one variable such as height is matched by a rise of 10% in the value of another such as weight) would have a correlation coefficient of 1.00. However, values of 0.6 or 0.7 can be indicators of a strong link. A minus sign in front of the figure suggests a negative relationship where as the value of one variable goes up the value of the other goes down (e.g. the longer someone has been qualified, the lower the level of anxiety when carrying out complex clinical procedures). The absence of a minus sign indicates a positive correlation, that is, as the value of one variable goes up, values in the other variable go up too (e.g. the longer someone has been qualified, the more frequently they include advice on health promoting activities when talking to patients).

See also: Statistics, data analysis.

Covert observation

Related to: Observation, research methods, tools of data collection.

Definition: A method of gathering observational data without the knowledge and consent of those being observed.

Application: A fundamental aspect of research data is its accuracy. The problem for the researcher is to gather the data as accurately as possible. Therefore, when collecting observational data, the more open the process of observation (overt observation), the higher the possibility that the individuals observed will change their behaviour and the accuracy of the results will be reduced. One solution is covert observation, where the process of observation is hidden from those observed in an attempt to ensure that they are behaving normally.

Key revision points: There is always a relationship between the research question and other aspects of a research study. Where the aim of the study relates to behaviour, observation is a potential research method to collect the data. Covert observation can seem a good method to reduce the possibility of inaccurate results through recalling what has happened in the past, but covert observation can lead to ethical issues such as informed consent. A balance has to be achieved between the quality of the data and the protection of those involved from abuses of their human rights. Ethics committees will usually support the individual's right not to be observed without their knowledge and consent, unless the level of possible harm from covert observation is negligible and attempts are made to gain consent for the use of the data retrospectively. This is not a commonly supported approach because of the sensitivity in relation to the ethical issues involved.

See also: Research designs, ethics.

Credibility

Related to: Qualitative research designs.

Definition: The confidence that we can have in the accuracy or 'truthfulness' of the findings of a qualitative study and the interpretation that the researcher makes from the data.

Application: As qualitative research is so different from quantitative research in the beliefs that researchers hold about the nature of research and the best way of conducting it, we need a different method of evaluating this type of study from that used with quantitative research. Credibility is one characteristic the researcher has to build into the report of their study to demonstrate that we can trust the results.

Key revision points: A frequently mentioned guide to assess qualitative research is the criteria developed by Lincoln and Guba (other references include Guba, as well as Guba and Lincoln which all cover similar points). In this material, the key issues relate to the concepts of *credibility, transferability, dependability and confirmability.* In essence, together these suggest that when reading a qualitative study you must feel that the data are genuine and that you can recognise the truth in what the researcher is describing. This is achieved through the author's use of descriptions that are described as rich 'thick' data, where the details almost transport you to the setting and you can 'see' the circumstances and environment and 'hear' the voices of those providing the data.

To achieve credibility, the researcher should spend time in the environment of the study and be in contact with the individuals to form 'prolonged engagement', which is likely to lead to respondents trusting the researcher enough to share valuable information. To build up the evidence of credibility, the researcher may ask respondents to look at transcripts of conversations and the researcher's interpretation of events to ensure that they are recognisable by those involved as part of a 'member's check' on the data. If there are clear indications of credibility, transferability, dependability and confirmability, then the researcher is said to have demonstrated the trustworthiness of the data.

See also: Transferability, dependability, confirmability, fittingness.

Cross-over design

Related to: Experimental designs.

Definition: An experimental design where one group of subjects act as their own control and are exposed to two or more interventions or situations in a study.

Application: One of the concerns of some experimental studies is that by taking two groups in the classic experimental and control group set-up, we are not controlling for differences in the personal make-up of those in the two groups. The crossover design overcomes this as it is the same group of people who experience both the experimental and the control interventions.

Key revision points: This approach is also called a 'within-subjects' approach as it is carried out on one group of people. Although the argument supporting individuals acting as their own control seems very plausible, it is fraught with difficulties. A major problem is that one intervention may continue to produce a response that lingers for some time, or only slowly emerges, and if introduced first as an intervention may be creating effects that might be mistaken for the results of the second intervention. This is called the 'carry-over effect'. This can be reduced to some extent by dividing the group into two and have each group receiving the interventions in a different order to ensure that the carry-over effect may be identified and controlled. The second method of controlling for this is to wait for some time before the second intervention. This is called the 'washout' period, which gives time for things to pass through the body or memory of the experience.

See also: Experimental design.

Cross-sectional study

Related to: Study design.

Definition: The collection of data, usually in a survey, from several groups or subgroups at a single point in time, rather than following one group through time as in a longitudinal study.

Application: In studies looking at changes over time, the researcher may follow one group over time and repeatedly collect data at strategic points, or collect data at one time period from different groups who are at varying points of experience or change. An example would be examining the development of a sense of professional responsibility in nursing students over a 3-year pre-registration course. The researcher could follow the same group over their 3 years, or take a sample of first, second and third year students and collect data from each group at one point of time.

Key revision points: A cross-sectional study would clearly be a great deal quicker and cheaper than a longitudinal study, but the limitation is that there is an assumption that each group is comparable and that no other factors affected their view of professional responsibility, for example, different lecturers, changes in course content or variations in clinical experiences. The cheaper cost of cross-sectional studies and the production of a speedier result still make them a very attractive research approach.

See also: Research design.

Critique (critique frameworks)

Related to: Critical assessment of published research.

Definition: Taking a balanced view of a research article focussing on methodological strengths and any limitations in order to come to some judgement on its merit and application to practice.

Application: Research should not be accepted on face value; it should be critically analysed in relation to the principles of research. There are several frameworks for critically analysing research articles. These can differ depending on the type of research evaluated. For example, qualitative research articles should be critically assessed using very different criteria from quantitative research. RCTs have very clear criteria that are used to assess their quality. Such frameworks are important to use if clinical decision making is to be influenced by research that guides the way to 'best' practice.

Key revision points: Critiquing a study does not mean simply criticising, that is, just being negative about a study. The balanced approach to analysis is crucial as it illustrates that you are aware of the difficulties inherent in carrying out research.

There are two aspects to critiquing research: the first is to answer the question 'what did they do?' and the second is to judge 'how well did they do it?' This second question relates to the extent to which the principles of research have been followed by the researcher. When asked to critique research, it is advisable to use a named critiquing method or structure. This name should be included in your work. Be sure to ensure that your 'voice' is heard in the analysis. The evaluation of a study should contain an assessment of issues such as reliability, validity, bias and rigour in quantitative research and credibility, transferability, dependability, confirmability, fittingness and rigour in qualitative research.

See also: Principles of research, reliability, validity, bias, rigour, credibility, transferability, dependability, confirmability, fittingness.

Data

Related to: Research process, statistical analysis.

Definition: Information collected in research that forms the basis of a study's results. Usually applied to describe numeric data in quantitative research.

Application: Any study gathers information to answer the research aim. In quantitative studies, this takes the form of numeric information that measures the variables in the study in some way or quantifies the amounts of some variables or characteristics. These numbers will be processed to make them easier to understand through summarising the data or subjecting it to statistical testing to provide some understanding of the situation.

Key revision points: In critiquing research, it is important to assess how accurately the measurements have been made (reliability) and if they form measures of the concept that is being examined (validity). The way in which the numbers have been processed and presented is also important as any errors in processing can lead to mistakes in interpretation.

Many people can find the analysis and presentation of numeric data difficult to understand and may even ignore the data presentation preferring to seek the researcher's explanations or conclusions. However, it is worth the effort of understanding how data are presented so that you can bring your own understanding to the results section. In many cases, it is not the data that are important but the interpretation of them. By the way, if you find the wording of the last few sentences a little strange, it is because 'data' is a plural noun although many people have always talked about it as if it was singular. In your research work, ensure that you use phrases such as 'the data were', not 'was' and 'the data are shown in tables' not the data 'is' shown in tables.

See also: Descriptive statistics, inferential statistics, levels of measurement.

Rapid Research Methods for Nurses, Midwives and Health Professionals,
First Edition. Colin Rees.
© 2016 John Wiley & Sons, Ltd. Published 2016 by John Wiley & Sons, Ltd.

Database

Related to: Reviewing the literature, literature search strategies.

Definition: Electronic location that stores digital details of articles. Sometimes, they may also store copies of articles, including research articles. These are the source of material for a literature review.

Application: Commonly used databases include CINAHL, Medline, British Nursing Index (BNI), Scopus, PsycINFO and Cochrane Database of Systematic Reviews. When using databases, a list of key words is needed to carry out a search. These words are usually those that form the main aspects of the study title or focus such as the dependent variable (outcome measure) and independent variable (intervention), along with the sample group examined. Synonyms and variations of these key words will also be used.

Key revision points: Databases are different from search engines such as Google Scholar as they maintain their own details of publications. Databases also use articles that come from 'peer-reviewed' journals, where studies are filtered first for quality prior to publication. This makes the information more trustworthy. In contrast, as search engines merely trawl the web and gather information from any sources that match the key words, the quality of this information is not as accurate or desirable. Assignments usually require you to name the databases you have used in searching for articles for your work, along with the key words, the range of years searched (timeframe), and sometimes the number of articles (hits) initially found. Searching more than one database is advisable as each database carries different sources of information. Keep a list of databases and key words when working on assignments for accurate inclusion in your work. Further suggestions for key words can be found on the first page of many articles under the heading 'key words'.

See also: Literature reviews.

Data saturation

Related to: Qualitative research methods, analysing qualitative data.

Definition: In a qualitative study, the point in data gathering when no new information or issue are uncovered and participants are repeating similar material already identified by others. This is taken as the point at which the researcher can stop gathering further data.

Application: In qualitative research, the researcher does not have a target number of people in mind to include in the study. Instead, the sample size is influenced by whether new ideas or issues continue to emerge from the data. Where it is felt that no new findings are emerging, the researcher will end the study concluding that data saturation has been reached.

Key revision points: Qualitative research differs in so many ways from quantitative research that it is like comparing two different sports with very different rules. It is worth being clear on some of these major differences so you can avoid criticising a study for something they are in fact doing correctly.
Data saturation explains why some qualitative studies have such small samples; it is because there were only a small number of different categories raised by the sample and the researcher terminated data collection once the same comments kept reappearing.

See also: Qualitative research, sampling.

Demographic data

Related to: Sample, research results, data analysis, bias.

Definition: Basic identifying characteristics of a sample that help the reader to picture the kind and range of people included in a study. This mainly consists of items such as age, gender, social class and education.

Application: The accuracy of the findings of a study can be influenced by a number of variables; including the characteristics of the sample themselves. The researcher will usually highlight some of the major demographic variables in their sample to demonstrate that they have achieved a reasonable representative sample. Sometimes, the demographic data will be linked to the outcome measures in order to check for any patterns between them. Traditionally, demographic data open the results section in order to provide the reader with a quick snapshot of those who took part in a study. This allows the reader to be more confident in the quality of the results.

Key revision points: When looking at the results section of a study, do pay close attention to any demographic data. Firstly, use the data to gain an impression of the study group and how far they match those typical of the wider group. Secondly, look for patterns in the outcomes that could be related to the characteristics of the sample. Commenting on this aspect shows your skill in searching for points the researcher may have missed, or not made explicit. You can use this section to acknowledge the rigour demonstrated by the researcher in achieving a representative sample, or for the way in which they have linked the demographic data to the outcomes.

See also: Generalisability, bias, sampling methods.

Dependent variable

Related to: Variables, randomised controlled trials (RCTs), outcome measures.

Definition: In an RCT the dependent variable is the outcome measure the researcher is trying to improve through an independent variable (the intervention).

Application: There can be one or more dependent variables in an RCT, and these form the main outcomes for the study. The purpose of RCTs is to demonstrate that the introduction of an intervention (the independent variable) has led to a more favourable outcome in the dependent variable, such as reduced temperature, reduced pain, increase in sleep and reduced level of infection, in comparison to an alternative intervention (the control variable).

Key revision points: Dependent variables often encapsulate the goal of the health professional – reduced temperature or increased hydration and so on, so the dependent variable is a major focus for assignment work. There are a number of other key research terms that a marker would expect to see included in discussions of the dependent variable; for example, a clear *concept definition* that defines the meaning of the term used to describe the dependent variable, such as 'door to needle time', and an *operational definition* that provides a way of measuring the variable, for example, some kind of scale or simply common units such as minutes. When comparing studies, these two aspects of the dependent variable should be examined to ensure that studies can be compared. Studies can be compared and combined, where relevant, if they have similar and compatible definitions and measurements for the dependent (and independent) variable. In order to judge the success of a study, check that there has been an improvement in the dependent variable.

See also: Independent variable, experimental design, concept definition, operational definition.

Descriptive statistics

Related to: Research results, data analysis, statistical analysis.

Definition: A part of statistical analysis that focusses on summarising the results of the study in the form of numbers. Frequently used techniques are measures of central tendency (averages), such as the mean, mode and median, and other calculations including standard deviation and range.

Application: Although many people find statistics to be a difficult area of knowledge, understanding a small number of these terms makes a big difference to your ability to read and talk about research reports in a very different and more advanced way. The researchers' task is to make the results of their study easy to understand so that the key points related to the aim can be understood and their implication for practice interpreted accurately. Descriptive statistics are a necessary part of presenting results so that meaningful comparisons can be made between groups within the study or comparisons made with similar studies.

Key revision points: Descriptive statistics are a way of painting a picture of those taking part in a study or of the results using simple statistical techniques. These include calculating what was typical within the group in the form of *measures of central tendency* and the spread of the values in the data.

The measurement of spread of the values includes the *range*, which is the highest and lowest value or number, and an indication of how close the elements in a study (people or things providing the measurements) were to the mean value in the form of the standard deviation.

See also: Statistical analysis, levels of measurement.

Double-blind study

Related to: *Randomised controlled studies, bias, accuracy of results.*

Definition: A technique used in RCTs to increase the accuracy of measurements by concealing if an individual is in the experimental or control group. This is sometimes referred to as 'masking'.

Application: As with all forms of research, the accuracy of the results in RCTs is crucial to its success. Studies have shown that if those taking part in such studies, or those collecting the data know who is in the experimental or control group, their behaviour, measurements and estimations can be subconsciously affected. For those providing care, their treatment of those in the study can also vary if they know to which group they have been allocated. 'Blinding' or 'masking' are methods of concealment where those involved do not know who is in which group. Double blinding is where neither the person taking part in the study or those involved in data collection know to which group the individual has been allocated; single blinding is where only one of the parties is unaware; this is usually the person taking part in the study, but it can be the data collector.

Key revision points: Double-blind studies are regarded as high quality in the hierarchy of evidence as they demonstrate rigour on the part of the researcher in trying to increase the accuracy of the data. A study will usually state if blinding or masking featured in the design and include details of how this was achieved.
In some health research studies, it is not possible to blind a participant as the intervention they receive cannot be disguised in any way. For example, in midwifery research it would not be possible to disguise whether a birth took place in water or in a bed. In such cases, it cannot be said that the researches have designed a weak study as it would not have been possible to achieve concealment in those taking part.

See also: Randomisation, experimental design, hierarchy of evidence.

Ethics

Related to: Research process, rigour.

Definition: The code of behaviour and moral values involved in carrying out research on humans (as well as human tissue) that are crucial to safeguarding the human rights and welfare of those involved.

Application: There are a large number of codes and guidelines related to carrying out research. These have been developed and refined to reinforce key obligations on researchers when planning and carrying out research involving human beings. These include the following:

- The Nuremberg code
- Declaration of Helsinki
- The Belmont Report
- Research ethics: RCN Guidance for Nurses.

In the more recent past, research governance has been introduced as a framework to further guide and support health staff in achieving high-quality ethical research.

Key revision points: Ethics in research should be stressed in assignment work as one of the most important parts of the research process. They should be valued, rigorously pursued and supported. All research involving humans must visibly demonstrate that it is ethically sound in protecting the human rights of individuals and not put them at unreasonable risk or coerce them to take part in a study. Individuals must also be fully aware that providing research data is not part of their treatment and they have the right to refuse to take part, or pull out of a study at any point.

Ethics in research follow many of the same principles as those related to professional health services activity and therefore will be familiar to those working in healthcare. The first duty of the researcher is to do no harm (non-maleficence) to those involved in a study. Under clinical governance, this includes ensuring that the researcher has the skills to carry out a study and is insured and supported by an organisation that would accept vicarious liability for any error or harm that accidentally happens to those taking part. The main ethical issues include the following:

- Beneficence (doing good through the research)
- Non-maleficence (avoiding harm)
- Obtaining informed consent to participation
- Anonymity, by ensuring names and identifying information are not included
- The safekeeping and protection of all written and digital data relating to individuals
- Justice, by treating everyone as human beings in the same way without favour or discrimination

Rapid Research Methods for Nurses, Midwives and Health Professionals,
First Edition. Colin Rees.
© 2016 John Wiley & Sons, Ltd. Published 2016 by John Wiley & Sons, Ltd.

Ethics (continued)

- Obtaining ethical permission to carry out a study through meeting all the obligations of research governance and a relevant ethics committee, such as a local research ethics committee (LREC) or, in America, an institutional review board (IRB).

A study has demonstrated 'ethical rigour' where the researcher and the research team/organisation have followed these principles, where required.

In assignment work, use a more elaborate terminology for ethical issues to demonstrate your knowledge, for example, 'beneficence' rather than 'doing good'.

See also: Ethics committee, anonymity, beneficence, confidentiality.

Ethics committee

Related to: Research process, ethics.

Definition: An independent body set up to assess if the design of a study reaches a sufficient standard to ensure that safeguards are in place to protect those taking part.

Application: In critically assessing any study, it is important to establish if it has received ethical approval from an appropriate source. In the United Kingdom, this is provided by an LREC and in America the corresponding body is an IRB. Both are designed to protect those who are the subject of research and ensure that research designs meet the highest ethical, and not just technical, standards. If educational resources such as students or lecturers are involved, a University Ethics Committee may also be involved.

Key revision points: In the world of research, any study starts with satisfying the principles of good research design through meeting the conditions laid down by research governance. This is demonstrated by completing and submitting a national online application form to gain approval for a study. Part of the process involves ensuring that ethical considerations are paramount in the study design and that appropriate ethical approval has been obtained.

It is the role of local research ethics organisations to carefully examine research proposals to ensure that those taking part in a study are not put in any danger and that the researchers have correctly risk-assessed the level of possible danger participants potentially face. Informed consent must be given by those taking part and this must be based on a clear understanding of the implications of participation (what will happen to them and any areas of risk as well as benefit). Anonymity must be provided to individuals and all identifying data collected must be kept securely.

Ethical issues are a complex area but in published research it is sufficient to note that ethical permission has been granted, because only if all the other ethical issues have been satisfactorily covered will permission be granted.

Do use the language of ethics such as beneficence and non-maleficence, which mean 'to do good' and 'to avoid doing harm' when including comments on ethical issues in assignments.

See also: Research process, anonymity, beneficence, ethics.

Ethnographic research

Related to: Qualitative research designs.

Definition: A type of qualitative study that explores the behaviour, beliefs and culture of different groups and subgroups within society. It looks at individuals in a variety of settings, including the workplace, community and hospital health settings.

Application: As with quantitative research, qualitative research takes a number of different forms. In ethnographic research, the researcher attempts to answer a question on how a group of people sharing a specific characteristic, such as cardiac patients, or community nurses, behave, interact or develop a clear belief system. The methods involved include a variety of techniques, but particularly observation and interviews, to describe what people do and why they do it, so that we can anticipate or understand their way of life, reactions and interactions. The purpose is to allow health staff to provide a more sensitive level of services and care.

Key revision points: All research approaches have distinct features and are judged as rigorous by the extent to which the researcher attempts to gather data as accurately as possible, in line with the main principles of the method. Ethnographic research developed from anthropology, where the main concern was to document patterned group behaviour of often exotic tribes, and to offer where possible, an explanation for the identified behaviour and customs. It has been a feature of health research for many years, and often includes participant and non-participant observation to highlight important insights into group behaviour of both staff and patients.

See also: Qualitative research designs, participant and non-participant observation.

Exclusion criteria

See: Inclusion and exclusion criteria

Experimental design

Related to: Quantitative research, randomised controlled trials (RCTs), cause-and-effect relationships.

Definition: A type of quantitative research that compares the outcome of an intervention between those who have been randomly allocated to an experimental and control group. The purpose of the study is to identify the existence of a possible cause-and-effect relationship between an independent (cause) and dependent (effect) variable.

Application: This type of research design is a major contributor to evidence-based practice and systematic reviews of the literature. Its success if influenced by its ability to reduce the likelihood of explaining differences between the experimental and control group measures of the dependent variable (the outcome measure) by anything other than the independent variable (intervention). Systematic reviews of the literature based on RCTs are considered to be at the top of the hierarchy of evidence.

Key revision points: The basic idea of an experimental design is that it tests the effect of the independent variable, which is the intervention, on the dependent variable or outcome. This can best be identified if the researcher takes a reasonably large group of 'subjects' (people or things) and randomly allocates them either to the experiment group, which is the one that gets the intervention being tested, or to the control group, which gets the usual or an alternative treatment.

Randomisation is a key attribute of studies that test the presence of a 'cause-and-effect' relationship accurately. This is because it ensures that each group receives a reasonably even mix of other factors that may influence the outcome, such as age and previous experiences. The researcher must be able to control for other variables that might also make a difference. Measurement of the outcome variable such as pain using a pain scale is usually carried out prior to interventions, as well as after the intervention. As the groups should be similar in all respects apart from the independent variable being tested, any differences between the two groups can only be due to that variable, and a cause and effect is established.

Researchers are cautious in saying they have 'proved' a relationship, as studies are rarely perfect; they are more inclined to say a cause-and-effect relationship has been demonstrated or indicated. Because of this, it is better to avoid saying 'proved' when talking or writing about research studies.

The three attributes of a 'true' experiment are as follows:

- Randomisation, usually through numbering subjects in a sampling frame (list) and using a system that will allocate who is going to be in which group using computer-generated random. In the case of prospective studies, this can be done in advance and the treatment allocated in numbered sealed envelopes kept in sequence.

- Manipulation, where the researcher is able to carry out a different intervention (or no intervention in the form of a placebo or by putting on a standard or 'normal' waiting list) with each group.

- Control, where the researcher ensures that other influences (independent variables) are reduced or controlled in some way.

There are a number of variations in the design of an experimental study but in healthcare the RCT, which is the one described in the preceding paragraphs, is perhaps the most familiar. The level of precision and objectivity found in such studies make them being highly valued in evidence-based practice. This is because they provide hard and objective information to inform clinical decisions about which interventions have more successful outcomes than others.

The strength of these studies lies in the statistical relationships found between the outcome measures of the two groups. This is indicated by the 'p value', which calculates the extent to which the findings could have happened by chance.

Experimental design (continued)

Understanding p values allows the reader to quickly identify those elements where relationships between variables or attributes in a study are unlikely to be explained merely by chance circumstances. Experimental studies are not fool proof and several threats to validity exist. These should be explored when reading such studies (see Validity). The size of the two groups and their representativeness of the group being examined also influence the interpretation of the findings. However, the strengths of experimental designs, particularly RCTs influence their use in systematic reviews of the literature, and ensure their position towards the top of the hierarchy of evidence.

See also: Ex post facto studies, hierarchy of evidence, manipulation, quasi-experimental studies, p values, validity.

Ex post facto studies

Related to: Experimental design, retrospective studies, research design.

Definition: A type of study design that examines relationships between two variables using data already generated to suggest a pattern or correlation between variables.

Application: RCTs cannot always be used as a method for searching for cause-and-effect relationships. This is because practical or ethical issues prevent their use. In such cases, the researcher uses data that have already been created using a *retrospective* design and considers subjects who were either exposed or not exposed to a key variable. For example, consider a study to examine the influence of active verses passive coping skills and their influence on levels of psychological distress in women 1 year after a diagnosis of breast cancer. In such a study, the researcher would start with a measure of the dependent variable – level of psychological distress. The data would be gathered retrospectively by identifying the levels of distress once the sample was divided into those with active or passive coping skills.

This kind of study uses correlation and establishes a pattern between variables; unlike an RCT, it cannot determine a cause-and-effect relationship as other influencing factors cannot be ruled out.

Key revision points: Not all questions can be answered using an RCT; sometimes a retrospective study such as an ex post facto study is the most suitable design. Ex post facto means 'after the fact', that is, the data are collected once the subject has been exposed to the possible independent variable in the past. This means that there are a number of characteristics of the RCT that are not present in such studies; there is no random allocation as people have already developed characteristics or behaviour that place them in one group or another, this means that there is no manipulation by the researcher influencing who is exposed to which independent variable, the researcher does not have control in the situation as it has already happened; therefore, the result can only be a correlation. However, such studies do point the way to possible actions that health staff may be able to influence, or encourage, and to improve outcomes.

See also: Experimental methods, manipulation, quasi-experimental designs, correlation.

Face validity

Related to: Tools of data collection, accuracy, critiquing research.

Definition: Method of assessing the content of a data collection or measuring tool, such as a questionnaire or assessment scale. Draft tools are examined by topic 'experts' and also compared with previous studies or clinical texts to ensure that the content 'looks right' and is relevant to the concept being measured.

Application: In quantitative research, it is crucial that the measuring tool collects or measures relevant aspects of the variable under study. Where tools such as questionnaires and scales are newly developed for a study and untested, it is important to gain some assurances that the tool is fit for purpose and will examine the core features of the topic. This is done in a number of ways, for example, by examining the literature for what has been included in previous studies or professional literature on the topic. The views of specialist and experts in the field can also be sought for confirmation that the content and wording are relevant. In other words, critical judgement is used to judge 'on the face of it', does the content look right?

Key revision points: Validity is concerned with being true to the essential nature of a concept or variable such as 'distress', 'depression' and 'pain', that forms the focus of a study. Such concepts are often recognised only by their indicators, such as unpleasant sensations in the body or feelings of panic or foreboding. The goal of the researcher is to ensure that the right indicators are included in the tool of data collection and that respondents recognise those aspects that give the concept meaning for them. Achieving face validity is the attempt to ensure that the tool of data collection does allow the researcher to be confident that the concept is being adequately captured by their study. Face validity may not be the most scientific or accurate test of content; however, in many cases, it is the best available. It is far more convincing if this is linked to other forms of assessment that are more objective and measurable.

See also: Tools of data collection, rigour.

Fieldwork diary

Related to: Qualitative research, data collection.

Definition: Journal kept by a researcher during a qualitative study, especially an ethnographic study. Its purpose is to capture events, thoughts and draft interpretations of the unfolding events, observations or interviews.

Application: Qualitative studies are a vast exploratory enterprise and require careful management of emerging ideas, data and interpretations. A fieldwork diary, sometimes referred to simply as a field diary, is one method used by the qualitative researcher to capture such ideas and emerging understandings that otherwise may be lost.

Key revision points: The mention of the use of a fieldwork diary (or field 'log' or 'journal') is an important aspect of judging the rigour of a qualitative ethnographic study where there is a prolonged and often intense relationship between the researcher and those in the study. The content of such a document can also demonstrate '*reflexivity*', where the researcher records their continued relationship with those in a study, and captures reflections on the researcher's impact, personality, background, past experiences and personal interests on the unfolding of events, ideas and people in the study. This allows the researcher and the reader of a published account to assess the extent to which the researcher may influence some of the events and ideas being recorded. It can also provide confirming data on some of the points and can also strengthen interpretations.

See also: Audit trail, confirmability.

Fieldwork

Related to: Qualitative research, data gathering.

Definition: In a qualitative study, term used to denote data gathering in a natural environment or setting.

Application: Much of the language of qualitative research draws a sharp contrast with that of quantitative research. Here, the term 'fieldwork' is an attempt to contrast the 'naturalistic' aspect of qualitative data gathering with the artificial and carefully controlled environment of the laboratory associated with experimental quantitative studies.

Key revision points: Assessing qualitative studies requires attention to the details of the processes and data gathering that took place in specific natural or real-life environments within the study. In the past, research was often seen as being conducted in a laboratory, whereas qualitative research developed a contrasting language of its own and locates its activities 'outside' the laboratory, hence the phrase 'in the field' meaning 'everyday settings where the sample were found'.

See also: Fieldwork diary, credibility, key informants.

Findings

Related to: Qualitative research, data collection, results.

Definition: A term often reserved for describing the data produced by qualitative tools of data collection.

Application: Research studies can be divided into quantitative studies that produce numbers and qualitative studies where the data are usually in the form of words. Traditionally, to make the distinction between the two types of study approaches, the section in the publication of a quantitative research following the methodology was called the results and the same section for a qualitative studies referred to as the findings. Unfortunately, this system has slipped somewhat and it is by no means a commonly followed principle.

Key revision points: In talking about research, it is important to try and use the correct terminology to show the depth of your understanding. When reading research, the language will often follow certain conventions related to the type of study described. As indicated earlier, the distinction between results and findings is no longer a safe indication of the type of study.

See also: Results, qualitative research.

Fittingness (also called transferability)

Related to: Qualitative research, critiquing qualitative studies, transferability.

Definition: The degree to which the findings from a qualitative study can be applied to, or 'fit', other situations. The term roughly corresponds to the concept of generalisability in quantitative research.

Application: Fittingness, or transferability, is a decision a reader makes about the findings of a qualitative study based on the author's depth of description in the study that would suggest that findings are not unique to the study location but may be found and applied elsewhere. If fittingness can be identified, then it achieves the major category of transferability, which is one of the four main criteria set by Lincoln and Guba as part of their framework for assessing qualitative studies.

Key revision points: Assessing qualitative studies requires a different vocabulary and different ideas on what makes a good study. Fittingness, or transferability, as it was later called by its originators, Lincoln and Guba, is used instead of generalisability. This is because qualitative research does not claim the same kind of accuracy from which generalisations can be made, as happens with quantitative studies; rather it seeks to produce general insights. However, there is little point in research if the knowledge produced relates only to the location in which they were produced. Fittingness, or transferability, is your judgement that the revelations of a qualitative study do fit other situations and may have implications for your own clinical area. The author of such studies will frequently make the case for the fittingness of the study, but you must consider the strength of this case.

See also: Credibility, transferability, confirmability, dependability, audit trail.

Focus group

Related to: Qualitative research, tools of data collection.

Definition: The use of one or more small groups of participants to generate data through the exploration of a topic of mutual concern or experience in a discussion setting.

Application: Individual interviews provide in-depth information in qualitative research, but sometimes being in a group setting can develop a greater level of depth and understanding through participants sharing experiences and beliefs. A number of groups can be held with anywhere between 3 and 10 or more individuals. The discussion is guided by a facilitator sometimes called a moderator who is often joined by the researcher observing proceedings and ensuring that the discussion is recorded.

Key revision points: Focus groups have become an increasingly popular method of conducting exploratory type research. They generate a great deal of qualitative data quickly, and can often stimulate a greater depth of analysis or exchange of ideas, experiences and behaviour compared with individual interviews. They can explore topics such as coping strategies amongst people with a chronic illness, ways of developing skills or decision making amongst nurses and are very versatile where the group setting can promote revealing and sharing information.

The economic aspects of this method should also be highlighted, as they make good use of time and resources. However, as with all methods of data collection, they also have disadvantages, including the risk of individuals being intimidated or led by others in the group and therefore being influenced in the extent and content of what they share. This makes demands on the facilitator or moderator to control the situation, so individuals do not dominate the group. The key is to promote a supportive atmosphere to encourage a sharing of experiences and self-disclosure. The amount and complexity of the discussion, in terms of who said what, makes analysis challenging, but not impossible. As with other qualitative methods, it is difficult to generalise from the findings, but focus groups are capable of providing insights into topics that can improve care.

See also: Interviews, qualitative research designs.

Forward chaining

Related to: Searching the literature, literature review, key words.

Definition: In reviewing the literature, the process of locating recent article references in databases by using 'cited by' and 'similar studies' as a way of finding more recent publications.

Application: Locating relevant literature for a literature review depends on a number of techniques that will reveal as many good quality studies as quickly as possible. Back chaining, an alternative technique that uses the references section of articles to find similar publications, has the disadvantage of taking the search further and further into the past; forward chaining is the alternative. It is carried out by taking advantage of suggestions in the database such as 'this article was cited by … ', or 'other references that might be of interest are … '. Following these suggestions will usually reveal more recent articles.

Key revision points: A good review of the literature should focus on sources of knowledge that are as recent as possible. Forward chaining is a productive technique to achieve this, and will ensure assignments are up to date and include modern sources of relevant evidence. When writing reviews, name the processes used to find material and refer specifically to back chaining and forward chaining where used.

See also: Back chaining, reviewing the literature.

Frequency distribution

Related to: Descriptive statistics, results.

Definition: The number of times an attribute or variable has been recorded within a study, for example, number of readmissions by type of chronic illness over a 12-month period.

Application: The researcher in quantitative research must count and then describe how often a characteristic or variable appeared in the study in a way that is easy to understand. This often takes the form of a table listing characteristics, events or categories and the number of occasions or 'frequency' that they appeared in the study.

Key revision points: A large part of the aim of a study will take the form of a numeric display of the results. Tables vary in what they present, so it is important to know what you are looking at and how to describe the kind of display used. Frequency just means 'count' or 'number of occasions' and answers the questions 'how often does this characteristic or variable occur?' As part of critical analysis, reflect on whether the frequency for specific items is more than, less than or exactly what we would expect? The frequency for one item may be compared with that of another factor or variables such as age, gender or other category. Calculating a frequency is a reasonably simple technique. The important question is 'so what?' How might this frequency be an important finding in the study and does it help answer the aim?

See also: Descriptive statistics, table, levels of measurement.

Generalisability

Related to: Quantitative research, critiquing, research utilisation.

Definition: The ability to confidently apply the results of a study to the wider relevant population or situation.

Application: Part of the characteristics of research is the production of knowledge that can be applied to other places beyond the location of a particular study. In other words, research knowledge should have a general, not unique, applicability or relevance.

Key revision points: In assessing a study, examine the nature of the sample and consider whether they can represent a wider group. The limitations, or weak areas, of a study will reduce the extent to which it is possible to generalise the findings. Has the researcher clearly followed the research process and produced a study that has reached a high standard? The more it is possible to confirm this, the more trust we can have in the generalisability of the work.

The generalisability of research is one of the defining characteristics that separates it from audit and practice development.

See also: Research process, bias, critique, rigour, sample.

Rapid Research Methods for Nurses, Midwives and Health Professionals,
First Edition. Colin Rees.
© 2016 John Wiley & Sons, Ltd. Published 2016 by John Wiley & Sons, Ltd.

Grey literature

Related to: Reviewing the literature.

Definition: The inclusion of unpublished work such as conference papers and dissertations/theses in a review of the literature, particularly, a systematic review of the literature.

Application: Reviews of the literature, especially systematic reviews, are built on recent, high-quality studies as these indicate 'state-of-the-art knowledge'. However, some important sources of knowledge may be as yet unpublished, but are available as conference papers and dissertations. Providing they are judged to reach a high standard and fit the inclusion and exclusion criteria of the study, they can be included in a review.

Key revision points: Grey literature provides the opportunity to consider including cutting edge recent research in a systematic review of the literature without waiting for it to be published and therefore it forms an important source of evidence. It is called 'grey' literature as it does not exist on the white paper of a publication at the point of use, so the term 'grey' was accepted as a generic term to describe it. Not all reviews will include it, as it can be difficult to access. As with published papers, where it has been included, the reader should look for assurances that it has been critically evaluated. Your coursework may not expect you to include grey literature, so do check.

See also: Literature review.

Grounded theory

Related to: Qualitative research designs.

Definition: Type of qualitative research design that not only describes a social situation but also attempts to suggest an explanation or theory to account for it. Its name derives from the aim of developing theories grounded or emerging from the data collected.

Application: This is one of the more popular qualitative designs used in healthcare. It can look like other designs but its focus on explanation and often the use of a theoretical framework makes it different from some of the more descriptive qualitative research designs.

Key revision points: This is not a quantitative theory testing approach but a qualitative theory generating activity. Grounded theory developed from the work of two American sociologists – Glaser and Strauss – in the 1960s. It is concerned with human behaviour, and the way it is built around solving problems within social life. Details of both the 'essential' nature of the problem and the patterned human behaviour in relation to it emerge from the data collected in an inductive process.

Grounded theory often makes use of triangulation, that is, the application of several forms of data collection, particularly observation and interviews, but often combined with other sources such as documents. As with all qualitative approaches, the emphasis is on the analysis of the findings, and this is often carried out alongside data collection. This parallel process of data collection and analysis has an effect on the size of the sample, as collection stops once 'data saturation' has been reached. It also affects what information is collected next. During analysis, new data are compared with data previously collected in a process called the constant comparative method.

There are many different views on how to conduct such studies and even Glaser and Strauss, the two originators, went their different ways and argued about the nature of grounded theory research. Most published studies will contain the words 'grounded theory' in the title or abstract.

See also: Phenomenology, ethnographic research, data saturation.

Hawthorne effect

Related to: Threats to validity, bias, experimental studies.

Definition: A change in participants' behaviour due to the excitement or novelty of taking part in a study, rather than the introduction of the independent variable under review.

Application: Accuracy of measurement is a key element in research where the outcome should be a reflection of the concept being measured (validity). However, there are a number of threats to such accuracy; one of them is the Hawthorne effect where subjects can act and report situations differently because they are in a study rather than as a direct result of an independent variable.

Key revision points: The term comes from a number of connected American experiments carried out in the 1920s and 1930s in the Western Electric Corporation Hawthorne plant near Chicago. The purpose of these studies was to examine environmental influences, such as lighting and heating, on worker productivity. It was found that workers increased their daily work output no matter what was changed in the working environment. The conclusion was that it was regular contact, interest and feedback from the research observers that increased productivity, rather than the environmental changes. The term is now used as a warning of the unintended effect on some participants of taking part in a study that can be mistaken for the influence of an experimental variable.

See also: Validity.

Rapid Research Methods for Nurses, Midwives and Health Professionals,
First Edition. Colin Rees.
© 2016 John Wiley & Sons, Ltd. Published 2016 by John Wiley & Sons, Ltd.

Hermeneutics

Related to: Phenomenology, qualitative research.

Definition: A type of phenomenological research where there is an attempt to understand and interpret the lived experience of those in the study and not just describe it.

Application: Qualitative research takes many forms; one of the frequently followed approaches is phenomenological research. This provides insights and understanding of how people live their lives and their beliefs in relation to health and illness issues. It includes research focussing on staff, patients and the public. As with many research approaches, there are a number of alternatives in the way such studies are conducted and hermeneutics is one of those variations.

Key revision points: Hermeneutics takes its name from Hermes, a character in Greek mythology, who was the winged messenger of the gods. He frequently found himself acting as a go-between delivering messages from the gods to the people below on earth over whom the gods ruled. However, as the common people had difficulty understanding the language of the gods Hermes had to attempt to interpret the content of messages. Hermeneutics, then, is concerned with looking at observed behaviour or interview transcripts and interpreting their possible meaning.

As a research approach, it has been influenced by the disciplines of both philosophy and psychology. There are some notable key figures whose guidelines are frequently mentioned in the research literature; the German philosopher Heidegger is one such major influence who has given his name to Heideggerian Hermeneutics. He believed that human life is basically an interpretative experience, and people are constantly trying to make sense of the life they live. The researcher's role is to stand in the shoes of those in a study in order to try to understand their interpretation and understanding of life events.

Another influential German philosopher was Gadamer. Gadamerian Hermeneutics encourages the researcher to interpret written material, such as interviews, by looking at the way the parts of the text influence the whole document, and vice versa. This takes the form of a continual back and forth system known as the hermeneutic circle.

See also: Phenomenology, qualitative research designs.

Heterogeneity and homogeneity

Related to: Sampling, generalisability, bias.

Definition: Heterogeneity is the existence of a wide variation in some characteristic or attribute within a sample, and homogeneity is the presence of a single form or variation of a characteristic within a sample.

Application: A frequent problem in research is achieving a study sample that reflects the composition of the wider population under examination so that the results of a study can be generalised to the population as a whole. Where the researcher has some control over who is included in a study (e.g. in non-experimental studies), they may choose the presence of either a wide variation in an attribute such as age or condition or wound site, or they may narrow the range in the characteristic of the sample to ensure that they are reasonably similar in some attribute. This is to reduce the number of variables that might influence the outcome being examined and make possible relationships between variables easier to identify. Each of these two alternatives has consequences for the findings and the ability to generalise from the results.

Key revision points: *Heterogeneous* samples show a wide variation in the attribute identified such as time since diagnosis or variations in educational background. This kind of a sample is more likely to mirror the range of variation in the population more closely, and so make generalisations easier. However, the variation in the characteristic may have influenced the outcome and so make certainty about its role on the outcome less clear.

Homogeneous samples will provide a group who are reasonably similar in attributes or characteristics that may have some influence on the outcome being examined. This will make it easier to compare different studies if the make-up of the samples is similar. An example would be to restrict a sample to only those with a certain grade of burn, or those who have been diagnosed with a chronic illness within a set time period, say the last 2 years. This would make samples comparable and rule out its variations as another possible influencing factor on the outcome. The disadvantage is that such samples limit the level of generalisability to only those with the attribute present in the sample, for example, diagnosed within the last 2 years.

As with many dilemmas in research, there is no clear winner and it is a matter of judgement on the part of the researcher as to which option they take.

See also: Sampling, bias.

Hierarchy of evidence

Related to: Utilisation of research findings, systematic reviews of the literature, evidence-based practice.

Definition: A guide to assessing the value or weight that should be given to sources of evidence in evidence-based practice. There are many examples of hierarchies but there is general agreement that the most valuable sources of evidence are systematic literature reviews and meta-analyses of randomised controlled trials (RCTs). These are followed by individual RCTs and then other options that reduce in value down to professional opinion or personal experience.

Application: Evidence-based practice is founded on a belief that clinical decision making should be based on research evidence, as it has the greatest degree of scientific accuracy. As more evidence is available than ever before, it is important to use the 'best' and most accurate sources to make clinical and service decisions. The hierarchy of evidence is such a guide and a number of versions can easily be found.

Key revision points: Evidence-based practice is a global approach to clinical decision making. It is concerned with applying the most successful interventions to clinical treatment contexts. There is consensus that the most appropriate source of evidence is research, and within that the RCT, as it compares one intervention with another, or against no intervention in the form of a placebo or place on a waiting list. The highly controlled design of RCTs makes them higher in accuracy than many other sources of evidence. However, as one study is rarely definitive, the top of the hierarchy, and, therefore, the most valuable source of evidence, is the systematic review that examines high-quality RCTs, and the meta-analysis that combines the results of several RCTs and applies statistic tests to the pooled data. Towards the lower end of the hierarchy are sources such as expert opinion as these are more variable in quality and the process involved in coming to a conclusion is not open to scrutiny as is the case with research and systematic reviews of the literature.

It is also worth emphasising that many health topics are still under-researched, so high-quality studies are not always available. In addition, some topics are not always suitable for RCTs because of ethical or practical issues, so the hierarchy of evidence provides a guide for other relevant sources of information.

It should also be stressed that the hierarchy is focussed on quantitative research, as it is the type of research most useful in examining measurable clinical outcomes, which are required to compare clinical interventions. However, professions such as nursing also require other types of evidence such as patient experiences and preferences, as part of the decision-making process. For this reason, it is important to acknowledge that this system works for certain health questions and problems but not all questions.

See also: Literature reviews, generalisability.

Histogram

Related to: Statistical analysis, forms of data presentation.

Definition: A block representation of the frequency of an attribute or variable that takes the form of continuous measurements from zero to a specified number.

Application: Results in a research study must be simplified and summarised in a way that does not lose the value of the results but at the same time conveys a clear understanding to the reader. A histogram is a line figure that allows continuous or 'ratio' data (which has an absolute zero below which there are no further measures) to be calculated and displayed.

Key revision points: Histograms and bar charts look very similar and therefore are easily confused. The difference is that the horizontal arm of the graph increases from zero in value along a scale allowing differences in the amount to be indicated by the position along the scale. The vertical bars touch to indicate this continuity, for example, time, age and temperature. In contrast, the bars of a bar chart do not touch as the concept measured cannot be divided numerically into smaller parts, for example, female/male. As such, the bars represent nominal or category data that can only be allocated into one attribute or another, for example, gender, type of equipment or the name of an item. The bars in bar charts can be rearranged in any order as there is not a progressive quality to what is being measured that affects their position in the 'line-up'. In contrast, it is impossible to rearrange the position of the bars in histograms as they are set in an increasing measurement of the variable (e.g. age, height) therefore altering the order of the bars in any other sequence does not make sense. This form of display allows a visual analysis of results.

Both bar groups and histograms have the figure number and title below the figure as figures are usually read from the bottom up (see Figure 2). This contrasts with tables, which are numbered and titled above the table, as tables are read from the top down.

See also: Bar charts, data analysis.

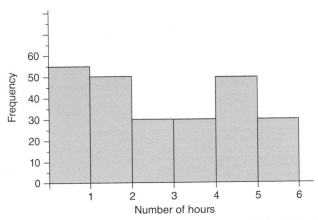

Figure 2   Number of hours of exercise per week by those who exercise weekly ($n = 239$).

Homogeneity (See: Heterogeneity and homogeneity)

Hypothesis

Related to: Randomised control trials, research questions.

Definition: A statement that predicts a relationship between an independent variable (intervention) and dependent variable (outcome). It is written prior to data collection and on completion of an experimental study the outcome data are used to accept or reject the hypothesis.

Application: A hypothesis is a traditional part of experimental methods where a researcher states what they expect to find when an independent variable is introduced and the effect it may have on a dependent variable. For example: 'the hypothesis of this study is that patients completing at least a one hour exercise period per day will have more uninterrupted hours of sleep per night, than those who do not exercise'. Here, number of uninterrupted hours of sleep is the dependent variable or outcome measure, and the exercise is the independent variable or intervention, no exercise is the control variable.

Key revision points: The purpose of a hypothesis is to test whether a cause-and-effect relationship can be demonstrated between an intervention and an outcome measure. There are three types of hypothesis:

1) Directional (also known as a one-tailed hypothesis). For example: 'there will be more/less of the dependent variable in the experimental group compared to the control group following the intervention (independent variable)'.

2) Non-directional (also known as a two-tailed hypothesis). For example: 'the independent variable will have an effect on the outcome measure in the two groups'. This form does not say whether this will result in an increase or decrease in the outcome measure, only that there will be a change.

3) Null hypothesis (also known as the hypothesis of no difference). For example: 'there will be no difference in the outcome measure between the two groups following the intervention (independent variable)'.

The null hypothesis comes from classical experiments where the hope is that the null hypothesis will be rejected, as this would mean that the alternative hypothesis, that there is a change as a result of the intervention, would have to be accepted. The null hypothesis is popular as any evidence of a difference means that the null hypothesis should be rejected. A directional or non-directional hypothesis is harder to accept as a difference between the groups does not mean that we can rule out that the difference is due to chance.

The acceptance or rejection of a hypothesis is decided through statistical calculations using a test of significance. This will state a 'p value' ('probability') that indicates the likelihood that the differences in results are due to chance rather than the independent variable.

There must be a hypothesis for each dependent variable in a study, so there may be several hypotheses.

Not all published experimental studies state a hypothesis, although it is very helpful when they do appear. However, it is not regarded as a point of criticism if a hypothesis is not included.

See also: Inferential statistics, experimental design, p values, dependent variables, independent variables.

Inclusion and exclusion criteria

Related to: Sampling, reviews of the literature.

Definition: Inclusion criteria identify the characteristics of the sample the researcher wants to include in the study so that generalisations can be made from the results. Exclusion criteria are those characteristics that may make the sample unrepresentative or endanger the health of the subjects if included.

The same principle is applied to the characteristics of a literature review where inclusion criteria states the kind of material the researcher plans to include in the review to ensure that it is based on representative and good quality literature. The exclusion criteria indicate material that could distort the findings of the review.

Application: In sampling, the problem for the researcher is to define before the study commences those people, events or things that will give the study credibility by matching the range of key characteristics in the broader population. The inclusion and exclusion criteria provide direction for the sampling stage of the research process, and allow those reading or listening to a study to understand who or what is represented by the results, and the decisions the researcher made to ensure that representative members were included.

Similarly, for reviews of the literature, the inclusion and exclusion criteria provide the transparency those critically evaluating a study should seek so that they can be confident in the rigour of the reviewer, and the representativeness and relevance of the material included.

Key revision points: One of the marks of both sampling and reviews of the literature is confirmation that the researcher has thought carefully about the characteristics of those people or publications to be included in a study or review. In both cases, the inclusion criteria should identify those who should be represented in the study if generalisations are to be made from the results. The exclusion criteria should identify those people or publications that might introduce bias. In the case of people, it is those who may be untypical, or those who may be put at risk through inclusion. In the case of literature, it is those publications that may be of a lower quality, belong to a different category or not really complement other forms of literature identified for inclusion. From a critiquing perspective, it is important to match the criteria against your expectations of whom or what should be included, and those people or articles it would be sensible to exclude in order to obtain a high-quality standard of work. In assignment works, it is worth highlighting your inclusion and exclusion criteria and your rationale for them where applicable and space permits.

See also: Sampling, literature review, critiquing, bias.

Inferential statistics

Related to: Quantitative research, statistical analysis, results.

Definition: A group of statistical techniques that allow possible relationships between variables in a study to be suggested or 'inferred' and evidence provided to support this.

Application: Inferential statistics are a group of statistical procedures that provide the researcher with possible confirmation that a statistical relationship exists between the variables under analysis. Some of the techniques may imply a *'correlation'* or pattern between variables, others allow a causal or 'cause-and-effect' relationship to be determined, depending on the nature of the study and the type of statistical technique used.

Key revision points: It is an advantage to have some understanding of how statistical techniques are applied to a quantitative research study. Briefly, there are two main categories of statistics: *descriptive statistics* that paint a picture of the findings of the study in numbers but do not suggest or confirm relationships between variables, and the stronger group of *inferential statistics* that allow a higher level of conclusion to be made. Inferential statistics include correlation, which suggest patterns or associations between two or more variables, and tests of significance, which indicate the likelihood of cause and effect relationships between variables. The latter suggest that one variable does have a change effect on another variable. Thus, an intervention (independent variable) can be shown in a randomised controlled trial to have a direct influence on an outcome (dependent variable) through the application of inferential statistics. For example, a study may test whether introducing higher levels of exercise on a weekly basis (independent variable) can have a direct effect on emotional stress levels (dependent variable).

The strength of these types of statistical techniques is that they indicate if the findings of a study can be applied more generally.

See also: Correlation, descriptive statistics, *p* values.

Independent variable

Related to: Quantitative research, randomised controlled trials, causal relationships.

Definition: The variable, or intervention, the researcher introduces in a study in order to measure its effect on a dependent variable or outcome measure.

Application: Research frequently takes the form of testing or establishing the influence of a clinical intervention on a key health outcome, such as the possible influence of levels of exercise on levels of emotional stress. In this example, levels of exercise and levels of emotional stress are both variables; level of exercise is the independent variable that can be introduced by the researchers and level of emotional stress is the dependent variable or outcome measure. The wording here is important as it is usual to indicate something is a variable, that is, it varies, by not saying the variable is 'exercise' or 'stress', but 'levels of exercise' and 'levels of emotional stress'. A study that looked at this subject would need to be a randomised controlled trial in order to rule out the influence of other variables, such as emotional problems prior to the study, and to suggest that differences in emotional stress levels have been influenced by the introduction of exercise rather than anything else.

Key revision points: Variables are the 'things' that vary in a study and an important part of the language of research found in published research. As nursing is committed to evidence-based practice, it needs a body of knowledge to support the use of successful clinical interventions. Much of this evidence comes from randomised controlled studies that highlight best practice in the form of independent variables (interventions) that can be shown to be most effective.

See also: Dependent variable, randomised controlled trials, inferential statistics.

Informed consent

Related to: Ethical research principles.

Definition: The agreement of an individual to take part in a research study based on a clear and detailed description of the study and the implications it may have for the individual.

Application: Under research governance, researchers must follow ethical guidelines including that of informed consent. This requires an individual to agree to take part in a study that is not an essential part of their treatment. The agreement should be free of coercion and given of the individual's own free will, having received a clear understanding of the implications of the participation. This should detail what they will be required to do or receive, and the possible benefits and risks of taking part. The researcher is usually required to demonstrate that informed consent has been gained in writing from the individual or, where relevant, from a proxy, such as next of kin or parent in the case of a child, who is able to make that judgement.

Key revision points: Part of critically evaluating a study is ensuring that ethical rigour can be identified. It is usually sufficient for a study to state that 'appropriate ethical approval was granted', as the role of ethics committee is to ensure that all ethical issues, including informed consent, have been identified by the researcher and addressed. The more invasive the intervention and the more vulnerable the individual, the greater is the importance of such issues as informed consent. This is more than simply saying 'yes' to take part is a study, the individual has to be given sufficient details about the study to allow a genuine decision to be made on whether to take part or not. Refusal to take part must have no repercussions for care, or anything else. If consent is given, it is not a once-and-for-all decision as an individual must have the right to withdraw from a study at any point without there being implications for their treatment or relationship with health services.

See also: Ethics committee.

Interval data (See: Levels of measurement)

Interviews

Related to: Research design, tools of data collection.

Definition: Person-to-person method of collecting research data using a verbal means of collecting responses to questions in person, telephone, online, or an instant messaging method.

Application: Data collection methods must be suitable for the research question, the sample and the type of data required. Interviews are suitable for extensive in-depth data gathering, where a study explores a broad topic or question, or where respondents are more likely to respond to a person-to-person method rather than a questionnaire. The form of questioning can range from a highly structured written list of questions, referred to as an interview schedule, to a more flexible list of key areas to cover, or even a single question 'can you tell me about ... ', followed by prompts for more detail where necessary. The form chosen will have implications for the type of analysis required.

Key revision points: Interviews are used in both quantitative and qualitative research studies. In quantitative studies, the data take the form of answers that are measurements, such as frequency of events, or numbers agreeing or disagreeing with statements, such as in a survey. In qualitative research, interviews are more unstructured and free-flowing, following an individual's experiences or thoughts. In this situation, their main advantages are depth and the ability to pursue new ideas or themes as they emerge, rather than simply following a list of questions.

The main disadvantages are the time taken to collect and analyse large amounts of often free-flowing data, the skills required of the researcher to avoid leading the individual in their answers, and the possibility that the answers are based on what respondents feel the researcher wants to hear, or the desire to appear a 'good person', also known as 'social desirability'. As with questionnaires, interviews share the problem of 'self-report' in that the data are not objectively gathered or confirmed; there is a reliance on a match between what an individual says they do, or has happened, and the events themselves.

See also: Questionnaires, quantitative research designs, qualitative research designs.

Inverse relationship (also called a negative relationship)

Related to: Statistical analysis, correlation, variables.

Definition: The direction of a statistical relationship between two variables, where as the value (amount) of one variable increases, the value of another linked variable decreases.

Application: In statistical analysis, there is a search for relationships between variables. Sometimes as the amount of one variable increases, another variable that is linked to it will also increase (positive relationship), for example, increase in physical exertion and heart rate, or as in the case of an inverse or negative relationship, the opposite can occur where as one variable increases in quantity, another decreases. For example, as the level of fitness increases, blood pressure decreases.

Key revision points: The direction of a relationship between variables is clearly important; the inverse or 'negative' relationship helps predict the outcome when certain elements are present in a situation. As this is a correlation, it is important to stress that this is a pattern commonly observed between variables and may not happen all the time, and it does not suggest a 'cause-and-effect' relationship between variables.

See also: Correlation, variables, statistical analysis.

Judgemental sample (See: Purposive sample)

Justice

Related to: Ethical principles, ethical rigour.

Definition: The ethical obligation to ensure that all participants in a study receive the same level of fairness and dignity, and are treated with equal care and courtesy.

Application: Accuracy is paramount in studies such as randomised controlled trials where there should be no influences on who is allocated to a particular group, hence random allocation. In the past, a number of studies were found to give preferential treatment to individuals on the basis of their social position or connections, whilst other studies involving hazardous interventions and treatments used only individuals from vulnerable groups. Some well documented studies also withheld known beneficial treatments from infected vulnerable groups in order to record the progress of certain diseases. The principle of justice is related to human rights and demands that in research everyone should receive the same dignity and respect of their human rights; all forms of discrimination must be avoided.

Key revision points: The concept of justice applies to the planning and implementation stages of research. It is part of ethical rigour, that is, the demonstration of high ethical standards in the conduct of a study. Other ethical issues include avoiding harm to participants, informed consent and confidentiality. In published studies, all these individual aspects are rarely highlighted although they may have been observed. Providing a study has been approved by an appropriate ethics committee, it can be assumed that such elements as justice have been examined by an ethics committee before granting permission to carry out the research. However, it is still important to ensure that from the author's own descriptions, participants' human rights have been protected and issues such as justice have not been compromised.

See also: Ethics committee.

Rapid Research Methods for Nurses, Midwives and Health Professionals,
First Edition. Colin Rees.
© 2016 John Wiley & Sons, Ltd. Published 2016 by John Wiley & Sons, Ltd.

Key informant

Related to: Qualitative research, data gathering.

Definition: In qualitative research, those people who provide particularly useful insights, knowledge or experiences relevant to the researcher. These individuals provide crucial information or help in accessing data that are beneficial to the aim of the study.

Application: Particularly, in ethnographic studies, where the researcher may lack a knowledge of 'the way things are' in a specific culture or setting, there will be people willing to share their expertise, knowledge or understanding to help the researcher understand the subtleties taking place.

Key revision points: Qualitative studies can place the researcher in unfamiliar situations with groups whose experiences may be very different from their own. Key informants can be very beneficial and lead the researcher to uncover the main findings quickly and efficiently. However, there can be disadvantages; key informants may have their own agenda, and their insights may not be shared by others in the same group. This situation may be hidden to the researcher who may be misled or find that other possible key informants do not emerge because of the association with individuals who are using the researcher for their own ends.

See also: Qualitative research, ethnographic research, fieldwork.

Rapid Research Methods for Nurses, Midwives and Health Professionals,
First Edition. Colin Rees.
© 2016 John Wiley & Sons, Ltd. Published 2016 by John Wiley & Sons, Ltd.

Key words

Related to: Searching the literature, search strategies, research articles.

Definition: Words used in searching databases and search engines to locate relevant articles for a literature review, also used on the opening page of some journal articles to indicate words or concepts associated with the article content.

Application: Key words need to be listed at the start of the process of conducting a literature review to give it shape and direction. The words are based on the main words found in the aim of the review.

A useful way of structuring the aim of a review is using the 'PICO' format, which stands for 'People/Patients', 'Intervention', 'Comparison intervention', and 'Outcome measure'. It is the combination of these key words that allows a potentially vast number of articles to be focussed down to those that will probably prove to be the most relevant. In a published article, these are often listed on the first page, or in a literature review, they are listed in the methodology section along with details such as the names of the databases accessed, the timeframe covered by the articles and any relevant inclusion and exclusion criteria used in selecting the material.

Key revision points: Key words that include the intervention, outcome measure and sample group allow you to find relevant articles for assignments and literature reviews quickly and efficiently. There is a skill to listing those words that will be productive. PICO can help; however, sometimes synonyms and alternative spellings are needed to trace relevant articles. Using back chaining and forward chaining is also helpful. The listing of key words is part of the transparency expected of a good article and similarly may be expected in a description of your search strategy for your review of the literature.

See also: Literature reviews, back chaining, forward chaining.

Levels of measurement

Related to: Statistics, data analysis.

Definition: Categorisation of numeric data into a hierarchy that indicates the complexity of statistical calculations that can be achieved using each level.

Application: In quantitative research, although 'numbers' may be thought of as a single entity, they fall into four different categories depending on the type of statistical calculations that are possible using them. The four categories are hierarchical with the bottom category (number 1 below) possessing little in the way of statistical function. The top one (number 4 below) is capable of the most sophisticated and complex calculations (Figure 3).

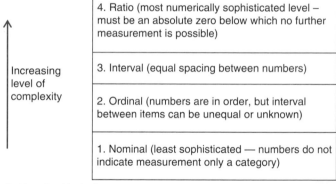

Figure 3   Hierarchy of levels of measurement.

Nominal data: These data use a number to represent a category label and do not measure anything. The numbers on the back of members of team sports such as football or rugby do not measure anything and so cannot be added, subtracted or divided to produce a meaningful result. In research, categories are sometimes allocated a number to make it easier to code or count, such as Female = 1, Male = 2. This illustrates that using some types of numbers in calculations is meaningless.

Ordinal data: These data are higher in the hierarchy than nominal as the numbers provide some kind of order, as well as allocate a category. Thus, runners crossing the finishing line of a race can be numbered with position 1, position 2, position 3. Although we know the order of who came where, the distance between each position can be variable and again restrict calculations.

Rapid Research Methods for Nurses, Midwives and Health Professionals,
First Edition. Colin Rees.
© 2016 John Wiley & Sons, Ltd. Published 2016 by John Wiley & Sons, Ltd.

Levels of measurement (continued)

Interval data: These data are the beginning of 'true' numbers as they measure amounts of a variable as the distance or interval between each number is the same, for example, temperature.

Ratio data: These data are the most sophisticated level of measurement, as they permit the most complex calculations. This is because numbers in this category have an 'absolute zero' below which it is not possible to have a measurement. While temperature does not always have an absolute zero as it is possible to have a minus figure (e.g. −3°), categories such as height or age do have an absolute zero as it is impossible to have someone with a height or age below zero.

Key revision points: Errors can be made unless the levels of measurement are taken into consideration. For example, it is not possible to calculate the mean (average) from nominal or ordinal data, but only from interval or ratio data. Usually, such errors will be identified prior to publication, but it is important to be able to understand why calculations with different levels of data vary.

See also: Descriptive statistics, inferential statistics.

Likert scale

Related to: Questionnaire design, attitude measurement, opinion measurement.

Definition: Method of structuring questions and their answers, usually in scaling techniques, questionnaires and interviews. Respondents are provided with a series of statements, called 'items', for which there is a list of fixed alternative answers. Often, there are five points (alternatives) to the scale but there can be four or seven points, although other numbers can also be found. Typically, these range from 'strongly agree' to 'strongly disagree' or similar structure.

Application: Likert scales are used to convert attitudes, opinions and views into a numeric value, usually ranging from 1 to 5 for each point on the scale in the case of a five-point scale. This provides a method of quantifying what is often thought of as abstract variable or personal opinion so that it can be subject to statistical analysis.

Key revision points: The Likert scale was developed by the American psychologist Rensis Likert, and so always has a capital 'L'. It has been a common feature of opinion and attitude survey research for many years. It is worth remembering that this is not an exact measurement and can be affected by 'social desirability', that is, individuals answering in such a way that they look the ideal or 'model' individual. However, it does provide a general idea that can be useful in the same way that a pain scale gives a useful indication of pain, but cannot be called an exact or accurate measurement.

See also: Scales, questionnaire design, quantitative research, social desirability.

Literature review (also called Review of the literature)

Related to: Research process, reviews of the literature, systematic reviews.

Definition: The critical analysis of a defined selection of available literature that answers a specific question.

Application: One of the important stages of the research process is to place a study within the context of current knowledge. This is achieved by carrying out a literature review examining relevant research already completed on the topic. This will inform the researcher on the current knowledge available on their topic and will form part of the review of the literature when their study is published so that readers can place their study in the context of previous work.

Literature reviews are also conducted as a stand-alone study that can inform practice and contribute to evidence-based practice. Such reviews are also a common feature of academic work and can take a number of forms; increasingly, however, a common requirement is that reviews should include the critical analysis of the research included and not just a summary or précis of the articles.

One specialised form of the review is the *systematic review of the literature*. These are produced by a team of writers to increase objectivity and avoid personal bias. The literature included in a systematic review has to satisfy stringent criteria to ensure its quality. The purpose of this kind of review is to produce guides for clinical practice that are sound and reach a high academic standard.

Key revision points: A good review of the literature consists of careful planning and an exhaustive process of locating (sourcing) the literature to ensure that conclusions are based on credible findings. They should demonstrate clear evidence of critical analysis to ensure that the limitations, as well as strengths of the literature, are recognised. Most reviews require the inclusion of details of the search process to meet the criteria of 'reproducibility'. This includes elements such as the databases and key terms used; the time frame, and inclusion and exclusion criteria used to assess the literature and the naming of the critical analysis framework used to assess its quality.

See also: Databases.

Manipulation

Related to: Experimental designs, randomised controlled trials.

Definition: The researcher's ability to control the presence or quantity of an independent variable in a randomised controlled trial. This is achieved by the ability to introduce the independent variable to only those in the experimental group and withhold or supply an alternative to the control group.

Application: In order to fulfil the criteria of a randomised controlled design, manipulation must be present to demonstrate that the researcher has been able to influence what happens within the study in relation to the independent variable (intervention) and limit the influence of chance circumstances.

Key revision points: The other two major criteria to be fulfilled in a randomised control trial along with *manipulation* are *control* and *randomisation*. Together these demonstrate that the researcher is able to achieve credible results that reduce the influence of other explanation for the results.

See also: *Experimental designs, randomisation.*

Masking (See: Blinding)

Rapid Research Methods for Nurses, Midwives and Health Professionals,
First Edition. Colin Rees.
© 2016 John Wiley & Sons, Ltd. Published 2016 by John Wiley & Sons, Ltd.

Measures of central tendency

Related to descriptive statistics: Statistical calculations, data analysis.

Definition: The calculation of a numeric value that indicates what is a typical value in a set of numbers. Although we typically talk about the average of a variable such as age, weight or height, there are several techniques that calculate 'average' in statistics. These include the mean, median and mode and together are referred to as measures of central tendency, that is, figures that tend to represent a value that comes towards the middle or centre of a group or 'data set' of numbers.

Application: In research, it is important to ensure that numeric results and ways of expressing them are clear and accurate. In descriptive statistics, measures of central tendency are used to summarise or describe what is 'typical' in a group of numbers and can take one of three different forms, each of which are calculated in a different way and may produce different results. These are as follows:

- Mean: This corresponds with our understanding of 'average' and is calculated by adding together the value of each 'unit' and dividing by the total number of units in the group (*data set*). As the value of the mean is influenced the presence of untypical values (or results) at either end of a data set, the mean can be distorted or biased by unusually small or large figures that will pull down or up the mean

- Median: This is a popular alternative to the mean, and is calculated by taking each individual value in the data set and putting them in order from the lowest to the highest. The median is the value of the middle number in the line of ranked figures and forms the mid-point at which 50% of the numbers are below the middle one and 50% are above it. In other words, it is the one in the middle of the distribution of numbers. If there is an even number of values in the data set, a line is drawn between the two at the mid-point, and these are then added together and divided by two to produce the median. This calculation is difficult to achieve manually if there is a large number of individual items in the data set. This is the most stable figure as it is unaffected by the size of the numbers at either end of the rank order; it stays in the middle regardless of the values.

- Mode: This is the value that occurs most frequently in the data set. However, this is not as stable as the median as it can be pulled up or down long distances just by adding a further unit that has the same value as other items that will make it the most frequently occurring value. This can happen at any point in the distribution.

Key revision points: Avoid talking about the 'average' of any quantity found in a study; instead, look closely at which measure of central tendency has been used, and use that wording. As with many ideas and concepts in research, there are advantages and disadvantages to each measure of central tendency, and it is a case of using the one that is clear and relevant for the intended purpose. The mean is frequently used in research, but because of its weakness of being influenced by untypically high or low numbers, it is often used in conjunction with the *standard deviation*, which is part of the measures of dispersion. Together these two techniques provide a better idea of where most values (or numbers) lie in a study.

See also: Data analysis, descriptive statistics, measures of dispersion.

Mean (See: Measures of central tendency)

Measures of dispersion

Related to: Statistical analysis, data analysis.

Definition: Calculations of how the values of a variable in a study are spread out, particularly in relation to the mean (see previous entry).

Application: In descriptive statistical analysis, the researcher will frequently provide an indication of not only how the measurements of an attribute or variable can be typified through a central or 'average' figure such as the *mean, median* or *mode*, but also how they differ in terms of their spread along a continuum. Here, calculations such as the *range*, which is the lowest and highest figure, *standard deviation*, how figures are arranged in relation to the mean and *variance*, which is a measure of variability or dispersion, which is calculated by squaring the figure for the standard deviation, are used.

Key revision points: The language of statistics is vast and built on a large number of principles; however, it is worth learning how to interpret and use some of the frequently used terms, as they help in understanding quantitative results and increase your ability to communicate a study's application to practice. Taken together, measures of central tendency and dispersion provide a numeric snapshot of the sample or results of a study.

See also: Inferential statistics, descriptive statistics, measures of central tendency.

Meta-analysis

Related to: Systematic reviews, reviews of the literature.

Definition: A type of review of the literature that combines together the numeric results from several studies, usually randomised controlled trials, to form a new merged data set. The reviewers then re-calculate the results to take advantage of the effect of a larger combined total sample.

Application: Individual studies can suffer from small sample sizes that restrict the accuracy of statistical procedures that require large samples. This can result in uncertainty on the effectiveness of treatments where the lack of a statistical relationship may be due to weak statistical relationships caused by a small sample size. Combining similar studies can overcome this problem and increase the accuracy of the results.

Key revision points: There are many benefits to pooling or merging data, such as an increase in the sensitivity and accuracy of the statistical processes used in such re-calculations. However, there are limitations to the use of a meta-analysis in that they require close similarities in things such as the same data collection tool, sample inclusion and exclusion criteria, as well as similarities in the type and amount of the interventions introduced. Look at these details in the methods section to ensure that it is safe to combine the studies involved.

See also: Literature reviews.

Mode (See: Measures of central tendency)

Median (See: Measures of central tendency)

Naturalistic research (See: Qualitative research design)

Non-maleficence

Related to: Ethics.

Definition: The obligation for researchers to avoid harm through their actions or omissions. Harm can not only be physical in nature but also include psychological, emotional or social harm.

Application: At the planning stage, the researcher must consider their study design and assess the potential for both positive outcomes (beneficence) as well as possible areas of harm. Although this is generally considered in terms of physical harm, even research designs such as the use of questionnaires can have a psychological or emotional impact through the recall of painful or unpleasant aspects of the individual's life or past experiences. Similarly, interventions and how and when they are carried out can have an impact on social life and routine.

Key revision points: Research must be carried out to a high ethical standard and the avoidance of harm is a priority for the researcher. In reading research articles, you may find that a study lacks details concerning all ethical issues, but providing a study has been approved by an appropriate ethical committee, it can be assumed that all key aspects will have been considered.

When you are discussing ethical issues in assignment work, using technical language, such as 'beneficence' and 'non-maleficence', creates a good impression of the standard of your work, as it demonstrates your knowledge and fluency in the correct language of research.

See also: *Ethics, ethics committee.*

Nominal data (See: Levels of measurement)

Non-probability sampling methods

Related to: *sampling, data analysis.*

Definition: Ways of choosing the sample for a study that do not allow the researcher to make unqualified generalisations of the results to the larger population.

Application: Although *probability sampling* methods, which include simple random and stratified sampling methods, provide a close approximation of what may be found in the larger population, non-probability methods, such as convenience sampling (also called opportunity or accidental sampling methods) and quota sampling, do not necessarily match situations outside the study. However, the methods are acceptable for exploratory research where the ability to be able to confidently generalise from the results is not an essential priority.

Key revision points: Where studies have used non-probability sampling methods, there is a limit to how far we can generalise the results. This is because it is unclear how far the sample matches those in the larger population. It is wise to see such studies simply as providing an indicator of what was found in one group or study, and be cautious over any extravagant claims by the author of any wide generalisations.

See also: Sampling methods, generalisability.

Normal distribution

Related to: Statistics, numeric results.

Definition: This describes the way some variables, such as blood pressure or body temperature, form a symmetrical distribution around the mean, where there is a similar number of items both above and below the mean. This is often described as forming a 'bell shape' because when the results are plotted or drawn on a graph the results appear similar to the outline of a church bell.

Application: The accuracy of some statistical calculations used in the analysis of results requires the results to follow a normal distribution pattern. If this is not the case, the results may not be accurate, and the interpretation of the results may not hold true.

Key revision points: The normal distribution is relevant to some studies that use 'parametric' tests, that is those numeric calculations and procedures that generate a high degree of precision. Where variables do not follow a normal distribution, non-parametric tests need to be used, and the accuracy of the calculations is less certain.

The extent to which variables in a study follow a normal distribution will influence the statistical calculations used. Each parametric test has a non-parametric equivalent, although their accuracy provides less certainty about being able to generalise the results to the larger group.

See also: Statistics, quantitative results.

Null hypothesis (See: Hypothesis testing)

Observation

Related to: Research methods, tools of data collection.

Definition: Type of data collection using visual methods such as human sight or film/digital recording. Observations can be structured or unstructured.

Application: Observation can be used in quantitative research where structured observation checklists can be used to count the occurrences seen or the types of a particular event observed, such as the number of people sat in a waiting area. Observational data can also be collected in qualitative research, where more in-depth information can be recorded over prolonged periods of time, for example, changes in hospital patients' behaviour when family visitors are present. Observation can be carried out in different ways by the researcher, for example, 'covert' data collection is hidden from those observed; in contrast, 'overt' observations are visible and open to the view of those observed. There are ethical issues of consent and 'harm' where covert observation is used, and, in contemporary healthcare research, this type of data collection is rarely used.

Key revision points: There are a number of ways of collecting research data, each with their own advantages and disadvantages. 'Self-report' methods such as questionnaires and interviews face the problem of reliance on the accuracy of what people say verbally or in writing. Observation differs in that the researcher sees for themselves what happens. However, if an individual or group know that they are being observed their behaviour may change and therefore inaccurate information may be recorded. This point illustrates the principle that bias and validity are built in to most methods of data collection. For this reason, it is important that we do not talk too strongly about research generating 'facts' or producing proof, but rather, that they produce indications and evidence to support suggestions and hypotheses.

See also: Questionnaires, interviews, qualitative research designs, quantitative research designs.

Rapid Research Methods for Nurses, Midwives and Health Professionals,
First Edition. Colin Rees.
© 2016 John Wiley & Sons, Ltd. Published 2016 by John Wiley & Sons, Ltd.

Observational designs

Related to: Research designs, non-experimental methods.

Definition: A general term used to describe studies where the researcher does not actively introduce an intervention, as in an experimental design. In observational studies, the researcher will observe situations and search for possible explanations on the development of, for instance, clinical outcomes.

Application: It is not always possible through practical or ethical barriers to set up experimental designs, such as randomised controlled trials, that involve the intervention of a researcher. Instead, the researcher may collect data by following one or more groups either *retrospectively* or *prospectively* and look for variables that may be responsible for differences in outcomes. The difficulty with this research approach is the lack of control over the influence of a variety of variables in the situation that might have influenced the outcomes.

Key revision points: Although the term observation is also used to describe a method or tool of data collection, here it is used to describe a research approach or design that does not use interventions or randomisation, as in many experimental designs. It is a term often used in medical literature to differentiate broadly between experimental and non-experimental studies. Such studies do not necessarily use observation methods as a way of collecting data (although of course they may do), it is simply a term that distinguishes whether the researcher intervened in a study with an intervention or whether they 'observed the situation' by collecting data but did not introduce a clinical intervention.

The common form of observations studies include the following:

- Cross-sectional surveys: collecting data at one point in time in the form of questionnaires or interviews.

- Longitudinal studies: collecting data by returning to those in the sample on a number of occasions over time to identify relevant changes.

- Cohort study, also called panel studies: following the progress of one group of respondents over time in terms of their progress in relation to a condition or treatment without a comparison group.

- Case–control study: where those with one intervention or condition are compared with another individual with similar characteristics but a different intervention or no intervention or different or no condition. These pairings are not randomly allocated to the two groups and neither is the intervention randomly allocated. Individuals are usually already receiving different clinical interventions and so naturally form two different groups.

All these alternatives are concerned with situations that are not manipulated or introduced as part of the study design. Some of these are retrospective, and look at situations that have already happened or treatments that have already been started in the past. Such studies can also follow groups of people prospectively through different decisions or intervention paths and examine the consequences of these on health outcomes.

The limitation of such studies is that they cannot confirm a cause-and-effect relationship, although a correlation may be possible. Statistical techniques comparing the different features in subgroups or comparisons between groups are used to try and strengthen the researcher's conclusions, but can never overcome the lack of randomisation, and the possibility of bias affecting the results.

See also: Descriptive research, bias, experimental studies, correlation, randomisation.

Open questions

Related to: Questionnaires, interviews.

Definition: Method of asking questions where the respondent answers in their own words, rather than choosing between a fixed list of alternatives provided by the researcher (closed questions).

Application: Open questions are used when it is important to record respondents' own views without influence or guidance from the researcher. They can be used in both qualitative studies and quantitative surveys to gain more detail, or where a list of alternatives cannot be easily constructed.

Key revision points: The choice of data collection method must provide the best fit in relation to the study aim. Where the aim of the study is to explore a topic and gain depth, open questions are used. This approach is more likely to result in a higher level of validity in the study, as respondents are not forced into choosing options that do not really describe or relate to their experiences or views. The disadvantage is that they require far more time and effort to analyse compared with closed questions, but the quality of the data frequently outweighs this limitation.

See also: Closed (closed-ended, fixed choice) questions.

Operational definition

Related to: Variables, critiquing, analysis.

Definition: The name or description of the method used to measure or quantify a key variable. It is the tool of data collection used to collect data and can take the form of a scale (e.g. pain scale, Likert scale) or standard measurement tool such as a blood pressure monitor.

Application: In quantitative studies, variables have to be measured in some way in order to produce a numeric value for use in statistical calculations. The researchers' statement of the operational definition indicates the way this has been achieved in a particular study. The type of measurement should be clearly stated in a study unless it is very obvious, for example, time.

Key revision points: Details on the operational definition for a key variable should be included in the details of a study. However, an author will rarely say 'the operational definition was ... ', rather they will include a statement such as 'pain was measured using a five point pain scale ... , etc.'.

As the operational definition reveals the tool of data collection, it should be assessed in terms of reliability, that is, the confidence you have in the accuracy of the tool. If you are producing a review of the literature, you need to be aware that different operational definitions may produce different numeric values, just as measurements in degrees Fahrenheit differ from measurements in degrees centigrade; thus, it will be difficult to combine or compare different studies that have used different operational definitions of the same concept.

The operational definition is related to the concept definition. The operational definition is the measurement of a variable, while the concept definition is the meaning or interpretation of the word as defined in a particular study.

See also: Concept definitions, Likert scale, reliability, variable.

Opportunity sample (See: Convenience sample)

Outliers

Related to: Statistics, quantitative results.

Definition: Numeric responses that are extreme or untypical in relation to the other responses or results in a set of data.

Application: In statistical calculations, 'averaged' results in the form of the mean can be distorted by the presence of a number of responses that are untypical. These may make the overall results inaccurate or misleading. These 'odd-ones-out' are sometimes excluded prior to final calculations, but it is usual for authors to draw attention to the presence of outliers in discussing or presenting the results.

Key revision points: In examining published studies, look at the spread of results in a table or figure and identify the presence of any responses that are a long way from most of the others and may be untypical. These may be well above or below the mean. Consider if these may affect the overall conclusion and look out for authors drawing attention to these responses, in an attempt to demonstrate rigour by alerting the reader to possible problems with the data.

See also: Measures of central tendency, statistics, bias, rigour.

Ordinal data (See: Levels of measurement)

p Values

Related to: Statistical analysis, inferential statistics.

Definition: '*p*' Values indicate the extent to which statistical relationships are indicated by the data in a quantitative study. The '*p*' stands for 'probability' that a relationship may exist.

Application: A major concern in quantitative research is to demonstrate the relationships between variables in the form of either cause-and-effect relationships or correlation. In the case of experimental designs, these can be identified statistically by comparing the outcome measures (e.g. pain or anxiety) between the experimental and control groups following an intervention to the experimental group, such as teaching individuals to use relaxation techniques. The problem for the researcher is that the measurements or scores for each group may be different, but may be explained by the role of pure chance and not the effect of the intervention. In other words, although the scores are different, they are not different enough to suggest that the outcomes have been influenced by the intervention.

In order to be more certain that the differences cannot just be explained away by chance, the researcher processes the data using one of a number of possible statistical tests of significance. The results, either in the text or in a table in a research article, will include a '*p* value', that is, the 'probability' that the results are likely to be due to chance. The less the results can be explained by chance, the more likely they are to be explained by the intervention used.

The following is a very simplified explanation of how to interpret *p* values so that you can look at tables in a more informed way. The three main benchmarks used to interpret *p* values are '$p < 0.05$', '$p < 0.01$', '$p < 0.001$'.

The first value of '$p < 0.05$' is commonly taken as the minimum value of '*p*', which indicates that the results are not due to chance but are due to the different interventions received by the groups. It suggests that if the study were repeated a large number of times, in less than 5 out of 100 studies, the differences would be simply due to chance. The rest of the time, if the *p* value was less than 0.05 then the intervention has made a difference. The further away the *p* value lies from 1.00, the less likely it is that the difference in the results between the groups is due to chance. In other words, the intervention is effective, and this gets more certain the smaller the *p* value. Thus, a value of '$p < 0.01$' is 'better' than a value of '$p < 0.05$' as it is smaller (0.01 is smaller than 0.05, and 0.001 is smaller than 0.01) and less likely to be explained by chance alone.

A more technical explanation is related to the use of the null hypothesis in randomised controlled trials where the researcher starts with the premise that both groups are the same; there is no difference between them. As indicated in the entry for 'hypothesis testing', the researcher hopes that data from the study will show that there is not enough support for this and the hypothesis will have to be rejected. This would mean that there is more evidence to suggest that the intervention has been successful. If the *p* value is less than 0.05, it means that the data suggest that the chances of supporting the null

Rapid Research Methods for Nurses, Midwives and Health Professionals,
First Edition. Colin Rees.
© 2016 John Wiley & Sons, Ltd. Published 2016 by John Wiley & Sons, Ltd.

p **Values** (continued)

hypothesis of no difference between the outcome measures in the groups is 5 in a 100 or 5%, which is not accepted as large enough to make it a safe conclusion that they are the same. In other words, there is a 95% level of probability that they are not the same. When it comes to a *p* value of less than 0.01, there is even less support for the null hypothesis that the results are the same for both groups, as there is only a 1% chance that they are the same. Therefore, once the *p* value reaches $p < 0.05$ or becomes smaller, such as $p < 0.01$, there is more likelihood that the results indicate that the intervention is working.

When used in relation to correlation studies, such as in survey data, the *p* value indicates whether there is a statistical support for a null hypothesis that there is no correlation between the variables being examined, such as a lower birth weight in babies where the mother is a smoker compared with those where the mother is not a smoker. *P* values of <0.05 and smaller show that a correlation does exist and the null hypothesis of no correlation can be rejected. It is important to state that correlation is not the same as cause and effect. It cannot be concluded that one causes the other, but only that they seem to go together, and that a pattern does seem to exist.

Key revision points: The ability to interpret *p* values is a valuable skill; it helps you understand quickly whether there is evidence to support an intervention or accept the presence of a correlation. Where a table includes a column of '*p* values', look down the column to quickly identify those situations where the *p* values indicate a clear difference between groups and where there is no difference between them.

The *p* values can also be found in surveys that compare two or more subgroups within the findings. In these studies, there is no randomisation and nothing has been introduced. In this context, the question is simply, are the groups similar in relation to some variable such as similar level of children with a low birthweight born to mothers who smoke compared with those who do not smoke?.

When used in relation to correlation, the *p* value suggests whether there is statistical support for the null hypothesis that there is no correlation between the variables being examined or whether there is a clear correlation present.

Table 1 summarises the main points to help you interpret various levels of '*p*' in experimental and correlation studies.

Note the use of '<', and '>' when displaying the *p* value. When the small end of the 'arrow head' faces the *p* ($p<$), it means 'less than' and when the large end is towards the *p* ($p>$) it means 'more than'. Anything more than, that is above, 0.05 is non-significant and has not indicated a good result; *p* values of around 0.06 are said to be 'approaching significance', but are taken still to provide weak support for the intervention. Only results where *p* is less than 0.05 ($p < 0.05$) indicate a good result. In some studies where accuracy of the conclusion is more crucial, the minimum *p* value is set at $p < 0.01$ rather than $p < 0.05$ so that the difference between the groups has to be greater and clearer.

It should be stressed that we are talking about a 'statistically significant difference' here, which has been demonstrated by the calculations. The *clinical difference* in the outcome between two interventions may still be unimportant, for example, heart rate or temperature may have been reduced by a statistically significant amount but the size of the reduction will not affect the individual's clinical recovery or health.

See also: Experimental studies, correlation, hypothesis testing, surveys descriptive statistics, inferential statistics.

Table 1 Interpretation of '*p* values' for experimental and correlation studies.

If *p* value is larger than 0.05 (*p* > 0.05)	If *p* value is smaller than 0.05 (*p* < 0.05)	If *p* < 0.01	If *p* < 0.001	If *p* is smaller than 0.001 (e.g. *p* < 0.000)
In correlation studies (e.g. surveys) that predict a pattern between variables in subgroups, the evidence does not support a correlation; there is no difference in the pattern between variables in the subgroups	Yes, there is a pattern between the variables demonstrating a correlation is present	Yes, there is a clear pattern between the variables supporting the presence of a correlation	Yes, there is a strong correlation between the variables	The strength of the correlation is even clearer
In experimental designs, the intervention did not make a difference to the outcome between groups; the results are non-significant (ns)	Yes, the intervention did make a difference to the outcomes of the groups	Yes, the intervention did make a clear difference to the outcomes and is well worth using	Yes, it made a big difference – there is a strong reason to use this intervention compared with others	Shows there is little doubt that the intervention does make a difference to the outcomes and is a better choice of intervention
For correlation studies, where *p* is larger than 0.05 (*p* > 0.05), there is no evidence of a correlation as variables are unrelated, with no pattern in variables by subgroup	In correlation studies, for *p* values indicated in each of the four columns above, a correlation has been supported by the results as the variables have been shown to follow a pattern that is unlikely to be the result of chance			
For experimental studies, as above	For experimental studies, as above: the smaller the figure (away from 0.05 to 0.000) the difference between the groups is unlikely to be explained by anything else but the intervention – that is the intervention 'works' and may be considered 'best practice'.			

Paradigm

Related to: Research approaches, beliefs of the researcher.

Definition: A way of seeing and understanding the world that influences the way an individual thinks and acts and can be thought of as an all embracing 'world view'.

Application: The two main paradigms in research are the quantitative and qualitative paradigms. Each paradigm supports different beliefs about the nature of research and the role and behaviour of the researcher. Knowing the distinctions between these two paradigms will clarify the variations found in the structure and presentation of research studies.

The two paradigms highlighted here are known by a variety of alternative names; quantitative research is also referred to as the *positivist paradigm* and is related to the belief that the purpose of research is the objective measurement of variables and the search for relationships between them. The role of the researcher in this paradigm is to ensure that they demonstrate objectivity and reduce the contamination of data through their own behaviour, prejudices or bias as far as possible.

The qualitative paradigm is also referred to as the *constructivist, naturalistic* or *interpretative paradigm*. This is radically different from the beliefs of the quantitative paradigm. Here, the purpose of research is seen as the exploration of the subjective world of individuals and the attempt to describe the world through their eyes. The role of the researcher in this paradigm demonstrates a higher level of interaction with the sample and there is a greater use of the researcher's interpersonal skills. There is also a greater degree of social closeness and equilibrium between the researcher and those in the study.

As each paradigm is conducted in often very different ways, it is not possible to critique one paradigm using the principles and criteria of the other. This may lead to dismissing a study that may be following the principles of one paradigm but contravening those of the other.

Key revision points: Academic success in many research courses is influenced by a grasp of the language of research, and the ideas behind those words. 'Paradigm' (pronounce 'para-dime' to rhyme with 'time') is one of those key words that you may be expected to understand and use fluently. A paradigm is often described as a 'world view' held by an individual as it colours everything they see; it can be compared with looking through different coloured sunglasses that give everything the viewer observes a coloured hue thanks to the colour of the lenses. In research, the choice of paradigm will influence not only the type of research and the form of the question a study examines, but also the role of the researcher within the study and the nature of the relationship between the researcher and those in the sample.

A paradigm is not simply a categorisation of research approaches; it provides an understanding of the researcher's beliefs about the nature of research, its purpose and how it is best conducted to arrive at 'the truth'.

In the quantitative paradigm, the truth is determined through research involving the objective measurement of variables, and the search for laws or theories that produce predictions on the relationship between variables and outcome measures.

In the qualitative paradigm, the truth is determined through the eyes of those involved in situations and described in their own words. There are no measurements or statistical calculations of relationships between variables; instead, it details experiences, understandings and interpretations. These may be in the form of descriptions, or perhaps explanations and 'theories' of what may be happening. The research processes, sample size, purpose of the research, the form and type of analysis are all very different from those of quantitative research and accord with the researcher's views and beliefs about the nature of research and the appropriate method of research activity.

See also: Research approach, quantitative research, qualitative research.

Phenomenology

Related to: Qualitative research, research design.

Definition: A type of qualitative research design that describes the 'lived' experience of people with specific characteristics or within the context of specific settings.

Application: Qualitative research comprises a number of different study designs, all with a common aim of building up a picture of how human groups see and live key aspects of their social world. Phenomenology is popular in healthcare as it examines how people experience or interpret a situation that influences their health or the health of others. This could be people or patients, in general, those with a specific condition or health staff themselves. The value of this approach is to give individuals a voice and allow staff to understand situations from their point of view.

Key revision points: Qualitative approaches have been often developed from other academic disciplines; here, phenomenology has been influenced by key thinkers in philosophy, such as Husserl, Heidegger and several others. Phenomenological studies attempt to discover the essential aspects or 'core essence' of a situation by looking at it through the eyes of those experiencing it. As with other forms of qualitative research, the data take the form of words and descriptions of the situation or experiences of those in the study.

There are several variations within phenomenological studies; for example, some follow the principles developed by Husserl and include the process of 'bracketing'. In these studies, the researcher sets aside their own experiences and beliefs to avoid contaminating the developing ideas and themes emerging in the data. In contrast, those following Heidegger, who was originally a student of Husserl, believe that bracketing is difficult if not impossible to achieve as well as unnecessary, rather, they believe it is helpful for the researcher to draw on their own experiences to guide the study. There are no right or wrong answers to this kind of difference of opinion, and research is full of such areas of controversy.

The critical examination of this type of research requires a different critique framework from quantitative research as the principles of qualitative research are very different. Similarly, combining studies from the qualitative paradigm in a literature review requires a different approach from combining studies from a quantitative paradigm.

Phenomenological studies have a great deal to offer nursing in providing a sensitive form of healthcare, and it is perhaps surprising that more such studies are not conducted within healthcare.

See also: Qualitative research, ethnographic research, grounded theory.

PICO (See: Key words)

Pilot study

Related to: Quantitative research designs.

Definition: A small-scale test of the tool of data collection to ensure that it will successfully collect the necessary data. During this process, consideration is given to the practical issues of conducting a study, respondent understanding of what they are asked to do, and methods of analysing data before starting the main part of a study.

Application: In quantitative research, the accuracy of the data gathered by the tool of data collection is a key issue. A pilot study provides the opportunity to try out the tool under realistic conditions in order to identify if any improvements need to be made and therefore ensure that it is fit for purpose. In the case of questionnaires and interviews, the accuracy of responses may be affected by the researcher's use of question wording, which may be unfamiliar or have different shades of meaning to respondents. These problem areas need to be identified at the pilot stage. It also allows the research team to ensure that practical issues such as overlong questioning, gaining access to carry out measurements, or developing appropriate ways of analysing and presenting results are taken into account.

Key revision points: The success of a study is influenced by many factors, some of which cannot be controlled; however, in quantitative research where there is an emphasis on the consistency and accuracy of the tool of data collection, it is possible to fine-tune the method used. This is achieved by using tools or measuring scales that have been used in previous studies, or if they are newly designed for a particular study, they can be tested in a pilot and any relevant corrective action taken. This is an indication of rigour in the design stage of a study. However, in quantitative research, the flexibility of the tool of data collection means that it may be continually changing, so a pilot study to ensure consistency is not required. There may still be a 'try-out' of interviews but this is not referred to as a pilot in the same sense as in quantitative research.

See also: Rigour, research design, reliability.

Population

Related to: Sampling, data collection.

Definition: The total group of people, things or events that form the focus of a study and about whom the authors seek to say something.

Application: All those in an identified population can rarely be included in a single study, so the researcher usually selects a sample from the population to provide data. The process of moving from a total population to a sample is full of complexities for the researcher, and the credibility of the study is frequently influenced by the size of the sample and the extent to which the researcher has been able to select a representative group to form the sample.

Key revision points: The population is not necessarily those who share a geographical location, but a characteristic of interest, for example, the population of people suffering lower back pain. In order to achieve a representative sample, the researcher must identify the inclusion (sometimes called eligibility) criteria and exclusion criteria that mark those in a study as representing the population.

When critically evaluating studies, the details of the sample should be closely examined to ensure that generalisations to the wider population are possible and that certain subgroups have not been omitted, or that those who make up the sample are not in a different ratio to those in the total population. Such situations will reduce the ability to generalise from the results. The match between sample and population, then, is a key factor in critically evaluating studies.

See also: Sampling methods, inclusion and exclusion criteria.

Power analysis

Related to: Quantitative research, sample size, statistical calculations.

Definition: Method of calculating the size of experimental and control groups in a randomised controlled trial. It is used so that statistical analysis of the results can accurately indicate real differences between the groups within a stated degree of confidence.

Application: A frequent problem for researchers when designing clinical trials is to achieve a sample size that will allow results to be generalised to the larger population. Power analysis is a useful method for calculating a sample size that will enhance the accuracy of the results.

Key revision points: Power analysis is a statistical formula to increase the accuracy of the results in a randomised controlled trial. Providing the numbers calculated for each group are achieved, its use will save money in avoiding larger and more costly sample sizes, while ensuring that the sample is large enough for the statistical analyses of the results to work. This form of sampling calculation is not relevant to other forms of study design.

When critically evaluating trials, compare the figures suggested by the power analysis against the actual sample size to give an indication of the strength of the statistical analysis. If the numbers in each group fall far below those suggested by the power statistic, the results will be less reliable than those equal to or above the suggested number.

Power analysis does not guarantee the accuracy of the results but they make it more likely within the stated margin of probability. They are another indicator of rigour in this kind of study.

See also: Experimental design, randomised controlled trials, sampling, rigour.

Pretest–posttest designs (See: Before and after designs)

Principles of research

Related to: *Research process, ethics, research design.*

Definition: The guiding elements on the design and conduct of a study that promote the safety of both researchers and those involved in research, and the accuracy of the results.

Application: Research is an expensive and time-consuming activity that must be carried out safely and accurately with a clear purpose and benefit. Although research includes so many different approaches, there are common principles that underpin all studies; these relate to ethical and methodological issues, and the competence of those carrying it out. They also relate to those organisations that commission and apply research to practice.

Key revision points: The following are some of the main principles followed by researchers. Research should

- be conducted safely following, where appropriate, ethical approval by an appropriate body;
- have the potential to provide benefit to individuals, organisations and increase understanding and knowledge on a topic or issue;
- be carried out by individuals who have sufficient research education, training, experience and appropriate supervision;
- store all data on individual in accordance with current data legislation and research governance guidelines relating to security and confidentiality of participants;
- where a study follows the quantitative paradigm, either describe a situation in numbers, or, in the case of an experimental or a correlation study, seek relationships between variables and move towards developing generalisations, and theoretical explanations. The results of such studies should be generalisable, that is, it should be possible to relate conclusions wider than the location where the study took place;
- where a study follows the qualitative paradigm, either seek to describe a situation in words or offer possible explanations, both of which should provide insights and increase the understanding and staff sensitivity towards patterns of human behaviour and experiences;
- have a clear rationale, aim or research questions and appropriate methods that will provide an answer to that aim/question;
- follow an approach to data gathering built on accuracy;
- provide a transparent account of the way a study was conducted and resulting data analysed;
- recognise aspects that could introduce or increase bias and reduce them as far as possible;
- follow a thorough and appropriate method of data analysis, where results are displayed and explained in ways that can be understood and examined by the reader;
- provide conclusion and recommendations that are based on and supported by the information produced;
- identify and highlight any limitations that might influence accuracy and the application of results or findings to practice;
- be communicated in an honest, transparent and accurate way so that others may learn from it, and be able to critically evaluate its contribution to current knowledge and its ability to guide or influence practice.

See also: Paradigm, research method, ethics.

Probability sampling methods (See: Sampling methods, non-probability sampling)

Prospective and retrospective study designs

Related to: Research design, data collection.

Definition: Features of a study where on its commencement the data required lie either in the future (prospective, e.g. randomised controlled study) or in the past (retrospective, e.g. ex post facto study, survey).

Application: At the planning stage, a researcher must design a study that will answer the aim or research question. For some questions, it is possible to design a study with the maximum control over the accuracy of the data and the conditions under which the data are generated by using a prospective study design. Such studies have strict quality control methods built into the method of data collection and allow regular checks to be carried out during data collection to ensure consistency in the quality of the data. However, this is not always possible on practical or ethical grounds, and data already existing have to be collected in the form of a *retrospective* study. In this situation, a researcher has less control over quality and accuracy, as data cannot be managed once created to the same extent as in prospective studies.

Key revision points: The prospective or retrospective design of a study is usually dictated by the research question and the practicalities of collecting data to answer it. The approach selected will have consequences for the accuracy of the data collected. As prospective studies have high levels of control, it is easier for the researcher to produce complete, consistent and objective data. Retrospective approaches run the risk of incomplete data or lack of detail that may be important. For example, methods that rely on memory or estimates of past frequencies, such as how many periods of nausea have been experienced in the last month, may also be less accurate than data gathered at the time of an event or intervention. Although prospective studies are a stronger source of data, it is not always possible to design such a study, and retrospective studies can be the only option.

See also: Study design, ethics.

Qualitative research designs (also called Naturalistic research)

Related to: Research approaches, research paradigms.

Definition: Qualitative studies follow a set of principles and beliefs about research that form a paradigm or world view. It focusses on the social world and its meaning as seen through the eyes of those involved. This differs in many ways from quantitative research approaches, particularly in relation to the presentation of the findings of the study, which are in word, rather than number form.

Application: Qualitative designs are numerous and include the more well-known phenomenology, ethnographic research and grounded theory approaches. Together, they offer a different way of structuring and analysing research studies. They have a particular affinity with nursing as they emphasise a holistic approach to answering research questions, and attempt to gain insights that can help thinking and action in relation to healthcare activities. Qualitative designs also value and provide a voice for individuals in contact with healthcare and those providing care.

Key revision points: Despite the large number of different research designs, qualitative approaches have in common a focus on seeing the world of health and healthcare through the eyes and experiences of the individuals involved. Almost all the stages in the research process in a qualitative study vary from those in a quantitative study as can be seen in Table 2. This indicates that the beliefs and actions of the qualitative researcher are very different from that of the quantitative researcher.

Although there are mainly clear differences highlighted in the table, the identical concerns of the final two rows should be stressed in assignment work.

There are increasing attempts to combine both paradigms in the same study to produce a mixed-method approach to research. Although this is not an easy amalgamation to achieve, using each approach at different points of a single study may be more successful.

See also: Paradigm, principles of research.

Rapid Research Methods for Nurses, Midwives and Health Professionals, First Edition. Colin Rees.

Table 2   Comparisons between quantitative and qualitative research.

Quantitative research	Qualitative research
Built on a principle of objectivity, measurement and precision in the production of numeric data, and where the researcher remains objective and detached from the data collection process	Built on the discovery of the subjective world of those providing the data, where an attempt is made to see the world through the eyes of those involved rather than those of the researcher. Findings are presented in the form of words. The researcher makes a more equal relationship with those in the study
The purpose of the research is to generalise the results to other situations and seek relationships between the measured variables in the study. There is a concern to establish laws and theories whose truth can be demonstrated through the data	There is no focus on generalising from a study but to produce insights and understanding that may be meaningful to readers. Some studies may result in a suggested theory or explanation
The approach to analysis is deductive; that is, the researcher starts with theories and principles and then collects data to see if the results support the theory	The approach to analysis is inductive where the researcher considers the data collected, and in a process similar to standing back from a collage, may attempt to suggest an overall pattern or picture that may explain the data
A comprehensive review of the literature is an essential part of developing the research question and important aspects of the methodology, particularly the tool of data collection	Although a general view of the literature may be gathered, there is an attempt to avoid an early critical review in case it contaminates the researcher's interpretation of the findings; interpretations of the data should emerge from the data itself and then may be supported by the literature
The research question is very specific and requires the collection of numeric data, which are processed statistically to reveal interpretations	The research question is broad and asked in a way that requires non-numeric data to answer it, usually in the form of words that are then analysed into broad themes
The tool of data collection must be demonstrated to accurately measure the study variables; hence reliability and the consistency of measurements are key concepts. Measuring instruments such as scales from previous studies or piloting of the tool before the main study are methods used to achieve this	The tool of data collection is flexible, as what is asked or observed may change as the study develops. There may be several separate data collection tools, such as interviews and observation. No numeric measurements are involved. There is little reason to standardise the tool of data collection so a pilot is not required, although there may be a testing of the approach or questions to ensure relevance to those participating
Data collection is extensive. Emphasis is placed on large sample sizes. Those included should be representative of those in the larger population to ensure accuracy of statistical procedures and the ability to generalise results	Data collection is intensive. Emphasis is placed on the depth of data. Those included in the sample should be individuals who have experienced or have relevant insights into the topic considered
Data collection and analysis are carried out in sequence	Data collection and analysis are carried out in parallel so that further data collection can take advantage of new issues and themes arising
Ethical concerns relating to those involved are major concerns	Ethical concerns relating to those involved are major concerns
Rigour of the research design and conduct of the researcher/team are major concerns	Rigour of the research design and conduct of the researcher/team are major concerns

Quantitative research designs

Related to: Research process, paradigms.

Definition: A way of structuring research studies that requires numeric data and the measurement of variables to answer a research question.

Application: In planning a research study, the researcher is influenced by the research question to choose a quantitative or qualitative design (see the previous entry on qualitative research designs for a comparison between the two designs). Once a decision on the design is made, it will influence almost every aspect of the study and therefore has to be chosen with care. The research question should indicate whether the answer will require numeric data and the researcher will then follow the path related to the quantitative or qualitative design selected.

The major subcategories in quantitative research include descriptive surveys, correlation surveys, experimental studies, such as randomised controlled trials, and quasi-experimental studies.

Key revision points: Often seen as the traditional 'scientific' approach to research, quantitative research designs are used in evidence-based practice to describe, measure and demonstrate frequencies (how often or how much of a variable is present), correlation or cause-and-effect relationships between variables.

Quantitative research is carried out using very different principles and guidelines in its construction and implementation compared with qualitative research. The same is true of critically evaluating or critiquing these two types of study for assignment work. It is important to be clear on the differences between the two designs, and what should be expected in the case of a quantitative study.

It is easy to confuse these two terms when typing or writing 'quantitative' and 'qualitative'. It is worth checking carefully that auto correction or a simple error in writing or typing has not taken place before submitting assignments as your marks could be affected if the marker feels you have confused these two.

See also: Experimental design, paradigm, quasi-experimental research, survey.

Quasi-experimental research

Related to: Experimental designs, quantitative research.

Definition: An experimental and control group design that lacks randomisation and is used when randomisation is not possible. The results can suggest a correlation but not a cause-and-effect relationship between variables.

Application: Although in experimental studies the use of randomisation is required to establish a cause-and-effect relationship, it is not always possible to achieve. An appropriate compromise is to use two existing groups, such as similar wards in different hospitals and use one as the experimental group with a specific intervention and use the other ward as the control. As individuals were not randomly allocated to the two locations, it is not possible to rule out some previously existing difference in the two settings that may have been responsible for any difference. However, it is possible statistically to identify whether a correlation exists between the dependent and independent variables.

Key revision points: The term 'quasi-experimental' means 'almost, but not completely', or, 'resembling' an experimental design. Such studies are also called 'non-equivalent control group pretest–posttest design studies', which gives a good indication of how they are carried out. The control group is also often referred to as the comparison group to indicate that a different situation exists from that of a randomised controlled group study. Such studies will usually state that it is not a true randomised controlled trial. The implication of this is that they are not as strong as a true experiment, which can indicate a cause-and-effect relationship. However, they can indicate the existence of a correlation between an intervention and a clinical outcome.

Research is about getting the best design to answer the research question and yet be realistic in terms of what is practical to carry out. The hierarchy of evidence places randomised controlled trials higher than quasi-experiments but the former are very difficult to carry out, and sometimes for a number of reasons, such as the difficulty of ethically allocating some individuals to a control group, a quasi-experimental design is used. Often the two groups in such studies will consist of those in two already existing groupings.

When critiquing quasi-experimental studies it is important to compare how similar the two groups were at the start of the study, if they are very similar (indicated by a p value of greater than 0.05, shown as $p > 0.05$, i.e. closer to 1.00) then it can be assumed that the two groups are similar and comparable. Any differences at the end of the study that cannot be explained by any other variable must be considered as due to what has been introduced to the experimental group and a correlation is indicated. In the same situation for a randomised control group, a cause-and-effect relationship would be accepted. It is clear that when writing about quasi-experimental studies you should stress that a causal relationship has not been found.

See also: Experimental design.

Questionnaires

Related to: Data collection, quantitative research designs, survey.

Definition: A method of collecting research data that consists of a list of questions where respondents fill in the answers themselves, often from a list of alternatives. This can take the form of a digital online questionnaire or paper copy.

Application: Often the best way to establish information from a person is to ask them. This can be in a verbal question-and-answer-situation as in an interview; however, a well-used method is to supply respondents with a digital or paper questionnaire they complete themselves. This is called a 'self-report' method. Questionnaires are used in surveys ranging from less than 50 respondents to 1000 or more. Questions can be 'open', that is, requiring a response written by the respondent in their own words, or 'closed questions', also called 'multiple-choice questions' that have a list of fixed alternative answers from which the respondent chooses. Fixed alternative answers are quick and easy to count and therefore cheaper to analyse.

Key revision points: UK studies use the word 'questionnaire' to indicate the tool of data collection; however, US studies often use the word questionnaire to mean a survey. As questionnaires frequently ask for personal experiences some people mistakenly believe that they are a qualitative method of research. However, it is the way the results are analysed and presented that determines the type of study. As questionnaire responses are added together and the results presented numerically, they are regarded as a form of quantitative study.

Similarly, although some questionnaires include open comments for respondents to add their own wording, it is felt that this indicates a mixed method. Again, this is not correct. Here, although there might be some qualitative data, it does not make it a qualitative study or a mixed-method study; it remains a quantitative study with some qualitative data.

Questionnaires have many advantages: they quickly provide data; they are cheap, easy to use and non-threatening for both respondents and researchers. However, they have many disadvantages, such as needing careful design and piloting to ensure that they are unambiguous and do not lead the respondent in ways that might bias the answers. The information can be superficial and there is difficulty in ensuring that the answers are accurate – a common problem with 'self-report' methods.

A serious and frequently encountered problem is a low number of responses to a questionnaire study. The lower the number of completed questionnaires returned, the less likely the results are to reflect the views and information of those sent a questionnaire. When critically evaluating studies using this method, search for the *response rate*, that is, the percentage of questionnaires returned. This can be disguised somewhat by giving the reader raw response figures, often broken down into different groupings, such as age groups and staff groups. Where this is the case, quickly work out the response rate yourself.

Questionnaires are a useful way of getting an insight into a situation, but can rarely be taken as any more than a simple indication.

See also: Survey, interviews.

Quota sampling (See: Sampling methods)

Randomisation (also called random allocation)

Related to: Sampling, randomised controlled trials (RCTs).

Definition: The process of distributing items/people in a sample to one or more groups, for example, experimental and control groups, in such a way that each item has an equal chance of being allocated to any one group. It is used to reduce the influences of variables that might affect the dependent variable other than the independent variable under study.

Application: This is an essential starting point for a clinical trial where the groups should be similar at the beginning of the trial before the independent variable or intervention is introduced. The purpose of random allocation is to decrease bias by reducing the role of the researcher or other factors in allocating who or what ends up in a particular group. It is quite an elaborate process and requires each person or unit to be listed in a *sampling frame* and given a number. Then, using a list of random numbers, either generated digitally or from a table of random numbers, a predetermined amount of numbers equalling the number required for one group are selected from the list of random numbers and the person or item that corresponds with each number in the sampling frame is entered into the chosen group. This is then repeated to allocate those to the other group.

In practice, where the total of those in the sampling frame will take part in the study, half will be selected using this process and allocated to one group and the remainder allocated to the other group. This system is very successful in producing a reasonably similar mix of characteristics that might make a difference to the outcome in each group. In other words, the system produces groups that should be on the whole very similar or 'homogeneous' in character.

Key revision points: One of the principles of research is that data should be collected in a way that minimises bias. In RCTs, it is the random allocation method that helps to reduce bias; its absence may never be completely guaranteed, but in most situations it is surprisingly successful.

In the situation of a prospective clinical RCT, where it is not known in advance who may be admitted for treatment and included in the study, the researcher uses sequentially numbered envelopes in which a treatment option is inserted. Who receives which treatment is determined using the random allocation system described earlier but using numbered envelopes instead of a sampling frame of individuals. The researcher inserts the appropriate treatment instruction in the envelopes in the sequence drawn by the random numbers. The envelopes are then kept in numeric order and each one opened as an individual consents to the trial and enters the research study. When each envelope is opened, those taking part have no idea into which group they will be allocated. In double blind studies, those providing the care may also be unaware of who is receiving what.

One word of caution relates to the use of 'random' in everyday use to suggest a system that is somewhat haphazard with little structure to it. This is very different from the process of random allocation in research, which is not in the least bit haphazard. Looking at

Randomisation (also called random allocation) (continued)

the description of sampling strategies, the method of *convenience, sampling*, also called *accidental* or *opportunity sampling* is closer to the haphazard system that people think of when using the word 'random'. As these two sampling approaches are frequently confused, it is worth ensuring that these differences are emphasised in your work.

See also: Sampling methods, heterogeneity and homogeneity, convenience sample.

Randomised controlled trials (RCTs) (See: Experimental design)

Range (See: Descriptive statistics)

Ratio data (See: Levels of measurement)

Reflexivity (See: Fieldwork diary)

Reliability

Related to: Critically assessing research reports, tool of data collection.

Definition: In a quantitative study, the ability of a tool of data collection to measure consistently and accurately.

Application: The reliability of a tool of data collection can be demonstrated in two ways, either by using a tool that is trusted and respected, such as one that has been used in previous studies, or by *piloting* the tool if it is newly developed. Sometimes, even a previously used tool will be piloted, particularly where it has been used in a different country or culture, or where adaptations have been made to it. In the case of a questionnaire, the researcher may also use a statistical technique called *Cronbach's alpha* that measures the internal consistency of the tool.

Key revision points: When critiquing quantitative research, reliability is one of the major evaluative concepts that should be used to ensure that a study is fit for purpose. It is used in conjunction with others concepts, such as *validity*, which examines if the researchers have measured what they set out to measure, *bias*, which is the amount to which distortions or negative elements may affect the data, and *rigour*, which is the extent to which the researcher has followed the principles of good methodological practice in carrying out the study. All of these contribute to ensuring that a study reaches a high standard and is capable of making a valuable contribution to decision making.

See also: Tool of data collection, validity, bias, rigour.

Research

Related to: Evidence-based practice, research principles.

Definition: A carefully conducted systematic process designed to collect data to answer a clear question. The processes used to produce the results must stand up to critical scrutiny, and these results should add to our knowledge and understanding of a topic or issue.

Application: Research has been carried out throughout history and across many academic and practical disciples. In healthcare, its purpose is to provide clear and accurate evidence to determine clinical care strategies. Although it is sometimes confused with audit and practice development, it differs from these in a number of ways; the main difference is that findings should be capable of being generalised to situations outside the site of the study, and add to current knowledge and understanding on a topic. Both audit and practice development are useful to local developments but do not necessarily transfer to similar situations, nor increase overall knowledge on a particular issue or concept.

Key revision points: Research provides the 'evidence' for 'evidence-based practice' and is now a major aspect of clinical decision making. It takes a wide variety of forms, each of which may vary in its methodological principles and approach to evaluation. The complexity of research and the vast challenges to its successful completion means that it must be carefully scrutinised. Most research will have its limitations as well as its strengths and these should be expected as a normal part of the process. A fundamental obligation is for all health professionals to have some understanding of research processes and the skill to critically evaluate relevant clinical studies.

See also: Audit, critique, paradigm, principles of research, research design, research method.

Research design

Related to: Research process.

Definition: The type of approach and structure used by a study to collect the data to answer the research question or aim. Designs can be categorised in different ways such as quantitative or qualitative designs.

Application: In the planning stage, the researcher must make a number of decisions that will influence the way a study is carried out. The research design is similar to a job description or blueprint that provides an action plan to follow.
Quantitative research designs include the following:

- Surveys (both longitudinal and cross-sectional)
- Correlation studies, for example, quasi-experimental studies, ex post facto studies, correlation surveys
- Experimental studies, including RCTs.

Qualitative research designs include a large number of options but the common ones include the following:

- Phenomenology
- Ethnographic
- Grounded theory.

These lists are not exhaustive. Each design has general principles the researcher will follow and may also have a number of alternatives within each one.

Key revision points: The naming of a research design is important as it demonstrates familiarly with the alternative ways of structuring a study. Where you are critiquing a particular design you should indicate any key features usually associated with that design and how they can be illustrated in the study and any deviations from the design noted.

See also: Paradigm, qualitative research, quantitative research, research process.

Research method

Related to: Research process, tool of data collection, data analysis.

Definition: The way in which data are collected and analysed in a study. The term is broader than simply the tool of data collection as it includes the processes involved in the way a tool is used or implemented, and the system of analysing the data collected by the tool.

Application: One of the valued principles in research is the transparency in the way the researcher explains the steps followed in carrying out the study. This provides evidence that a systematic, clear and accurate process has been followed. The method used should be in line with the approved or recognised ways of carrying out a research study. In assessing research, it is not the results or findings that form the focus of critical analysis but the methods used that will indicate if the study is fit for purpose. The methods or methodology section of a published study will provide the information needed.

Key revision points: Most definitions of research include reference to the systematic way that it is carried out; details of the research method form part of the visible ways the researcher demonstrates how they have achieved this principle. There are a number of research methods used in research that are usually associated with the two main paradigms. Table 3 shows that some methods appear under both headings but will take a different form.

Each method has clear principles that should be followed in its use and each has its advantages and disadvantages. The methods used should be appropriate to the research aim or question and the sample in the study.

See also: Data analysis, paradigms, questionnaires, observation, interviews.

Table 3   Frequently used research methods within paradigms.

Paradigm	Quantitative	Qualitative
Research methods frequently used within each paradigm	Questionnaires Assessment scales Interviews (numeric or mixed data) Observation (numeric data) Documentary sources, for example, records (numeric data)	Interviews (words as data) Observation (descriptions in words) Documentary sources, for example, diaries (providing descriptions) Triangulation (combination of methods)

Response rate (See: Questionnaires)

Retrospective study (See: Prospective study, case–control study, ex post facto study)

Review of the literature (See: Literature review)

Rigour

Related to: Critiquing research, research process.

Definition: The researcher's attempt to reach a high standard in the quality of their work by ensuring that problems associated with the method are identified at the planning and implementation stage and as far as possible reduced.

Application: The essential quality of research is that it should be conducted in a systematic and logical way that ensures the study reaches a high standard of accuracy. Rigour is demonstrated through examples of how the researcher uses knowledge of research principles, processes, dilemmas and methodological problems, and makes practical efforts to reduce them at the design and implementation stages.

Key revision points: Rigour demonstrates the researcher's attention to detail in relation to the aspects of a study that make a big difference to the accuracy of the results and the overall quality of the work. Demonstrate your skill in critical analysis when completing assignments and talking about research by including reference to the concepts of rigour, reliability, validity and bias. Your knowledge of these issues and your ability to illustrate your points with evidence demonstrates a clear understanding of research. Make good use of these terms as they all show your emphasis on the quality of research and the methods that create it and not simply a focus on the research results.

See also: Critique, reliability, validity, bias.

Sample (See: Sampling methods)

Sampling methods (also called sampling plan or sampling strategy)

Related to: Research process, sample.

Definition: Alternative ways of drawing and selecting the people, objects or events that form the source of data in a study.

Application: Data can be collected from people, objects or events. As it is rarely possible to gather data from a complete population, results are normally based on a sample or part of that population. The sampling method is the design of the process that brings those selected into a study and should ensure that they are as representative of the total group as possible.

Key revision points: There are two main divisions of sampling methods: *probability sampling methods* that produce a sample as close in characteristics to the total population as possible, and *non-probability sampling methods* where it is not possible to be sure how closely those drawn into the study are typical of the population. Such samples are not necessarily incorrect or of little use, it is just it is not possible to say how representative they are.

Probability sampling methods include a number of alternatives under the heading of *random sampling* methods, which are as follows:

- Simple random sample: where everyone has an equal chance of inclusion into a study from an identified target population. Random allocation is slightly different and applies to how people are allocated to the experimental or control group in randomised controlled trials so that everyone has an equal chance of being in either group. This is important to reduce the element of bias that might be built into the composition of each group. Such samples require a *sampling frame*, which is a list of all those who could be included. These are then given a number and a set of computer-generated random numbers or table of random numbers is used that lead to those names corresponding to the random numbers being selected for inclusion in the study, or allocated to a specific group. The main strength of this system is that it is not known before matching the names with the numbers who has been drawn for selection into which group, so there is no possibility of pre-knowledge that might influence who goes where.

- Stratified random sample: This is a variation of the simple random sample where sample units are divided first into appropriate groups or separate sampling frames, such as type/category/age/condition/gender. Representatives are then randomly selected from each of the strata or groups, using randomly generated numbers (see simple random sampling).

- Proportionate sampling: As in the last category, but the proportion from each group is in line with the proportion found in the population as a whole.

Sampling methods (also called sampling plan or sampling strategy) (continued)

- **Cluster sampling:** This method is used when it is not possible to construct a sampling frame of all those who could be included or when it is necessary to draw the sample from a large area. The sampling is carried out in stages with larger units such as regions or areas drawn first, and then working down to smaller units such as health areas, hospitals and clinical areas. Each stage consists of a sampling frame at that level and a selection process with the use of random numbers. Once the smaller units have been reached, such as a clinical speciality in a number of geographical areas, then all those eligible in that smaller unit or 'cluster' are included. This still follows the principle of randomisation but overcomes the problem of selecting from wide-based areas. However, there can be problems in that those at the final stage may share common characteristics because they are in close proximity to each other. This illustrates that throughout the research the researcher is faced with achieving a balance between advantages and disadvantages associated with practical solutions. Knowledge of these kinds of 'trade-off' decisions is important in demonstrating your knowledge of the complex issues inherent in the research process.

This group of probability sampling methods permit the use of a wider range and more sophisticated forms of statistical analysis that have a high level of accuracy associated with them compared with the next category. The prime ingredients include a sampling frame where potential 'units' are first listed and then numbered, a predetermined quantity of numbers chosen from a computer list of randomly generated numbers (or table of random numbers), and a matching process of those corresponding to the numbers in the sampling frame who are then entered into the study or specific groups.

Non-probability sampling: These sampling methods are simpler and cheaper to use but do not have the same level of accuracy in the results, as only more basic statistical tests can be used on them. These methods include the following:

- **Opportunity sample:** also called a *convenience* or *accidental* sample. Here, those units or people easily accessible are included on the assumption that they are typical. This form of sampling is sometimes confused with, and thought to be, a 'random' sample as there appears to be little influence on their selection, that is, they are picked 'at random'. However, this is not the same idea or process involved in a true random approach. As indicated in the last section, a random sample is very carefully sourced, and has a lower chance of bias than this kind of 'accidental' sample.

- **Quota sample:** similar to a stratified sample where a set amount or 'quota' of people from identified subgroups is included, but without the use of a sampling frame. This is a refinement of the previous opportunity sample that results in a sample composition that mimics the kind of categories and proportions found in the larger population.

- **Purposive sample also called judgemental sample:** where the researcher hand-picks those involved on the basis of criteria that might ensure that a wide selection of commonly found criteria will be included and therefore match the larger population more closely. It sounds like there could be a large element of bias in such a carefully selected sample, but the opposite is more likely, as it produces a closer representative cross-section for inclusion.

- **Snowball sample, also called a chain, nominated or network sample:** used where it is difficult to find ideal respondents because they are not clearly visible. Any that are found are asked to 'nominate' or suggest others who might be eligible for inclusion. Often used in qualitative studies, this is a practical way of solving the

Sampling methods (also called sampling plan or sampling strategy) (continued)

problem of recruiting difficult-to-identify or 'hidden' groups of people, for example, illegal drug takers. This method is open to the problem of a poor mix or range of characteristics, as people who know each other may not be typical of those who are more isolated and may have a number of characteristics in common. The term illustrates the way the sample starts small, and like a snowball rolling down a hill, gathers size and momentum.

When critically evaluating studies, it is important to ensure that the principle of matching the method of sampling with the research aim and design is followed, as this will reduce the possibility of bias and increase the relevance of the results.

In quantitative research, especially randomised controlled studies, there is a drive to achieve as large a sample size as possible to increase the chances of accuracy, and results that can be generalised. This tends to promote the use of probability sampling methods. In qualitative studies where the search is for those who have experienced some issue and the drive is not for exact measurements, the sampling strategies are usually non-probability methods. In qualitative designs, sample size is often influenced by data saturation, that is, data collection is stopped when no new categories or information seems to be emerging. As a result sample size is often small, but the compensation is a greater depth in the findings.

See also: Cluster sample, research design, data saturation.

Sampling frame (See: Sampling methods, cluster sample)

Self-report (See: Interviews)

Snowball sample (See: Sampling methods, qualitative research)

Social desirability (See: Interviews)

Statistical analysis (See: Descriptive statistics, inferential statistics)

Survey

Related to: Research approach, quantitative research.

Definition: A descriptive research approach that collects data from a large number of people.

Application: Quantitative research can be used to collect numeric information that describes a situation in numbers. The main research methods, or tools of data collection, include questionnaires and interviews. The questionnaires can take the form of paper or digital copies. Surveys are a popular way of obtaining a snapshot of a current situation. Survey data may also be used to search for a correlation between variables, for example, establishing if people who often exercise have a lower level of depression. Sample size in surveys tends to be large in order to include a good cross-section of those who represent variations in the larger population.

Key revision points: Surveys have a long history of providing useful information on a wide variety of health topics. The strength of this method is their scope, which has increased in recent years with the use of the web to collect data. However, as with all research designs, the researcher's skills in the design and implementation of a survey are crucial to the accuracy and usefulness of the results.

When critiquing, look for rigour in the design and content of the questionnaire; has it been used in previous studies, or if this was a specially designed questionnaire, was there a pilot prior to the main study? Consider whether the researcher has gained a representative sample and whether there is a good response rate. Has the methods/methodology section of a study given you confidence that the sample is representative of the larger population? Are the conclusions clearly supported by the survey results?

Although questionnaires are often considered as a cheap method of collecting data, large-scale surveys involving complicated analysis and interpretation can be costly. If effort is not to be wasted, the researcher must be clear at the outset on the purpose of the study and how the results should be analysed and presented.

Importantly, American studies sometimes use the word 'survey' to mean a questionnaire, whereas UK studies use the term survey to mean the research approach and questionnaire to refer to the research method or tool of data collection.

See also: Questionnaires, correlation, research design.

Systematic reviews of the literature (See: Literature review)

Table

Related to: Data presentation, statistics.

Definition: A visual summary of usually numeric data, mainly used in a quantitative study, such as a survey or randomised controlled study. Words can also be exclusively shown in a table where the usual structure of rows and columns is applied. If there is only one square or 'cell' with words, it is usually called a box.

Application: Numeric tables can take several forms from the 'two by two' (2×2) table with two rows and two columns to multiple columns and rows. These are referred to as a cross-tabulation or contingency table. These illustrate the results of one variable, for example, gender, divided into or 'cross-tabulated' by a further variable, for example, taking more than 30 minutes exercise a week. The format is known as a 'cross-tabulation' as it is one variable 'crossed' with another (see example later).

Each table should be numbered and have a title that describes the contents. Columns and rows should also be clearly labelled so that it is possible to understand what is shown. Often the squares or cells contain two sets of numbers: one is the actual number and the other, frequently in brackets, is the equivalent percentage (Table 4).

Key revision points: Tables and other visual presentations can be ignored by many readers of research reports, perhaps because they feel intimidated by the use of numbers, or are unfamiliar with how to read a numeric table. However, the critical evaluation of published studies should include time spent on each table to discover for yourself the story they tell. Every table and figure should be referred to in the text with some kind of comment on it made by the author. A good study will provide an interpretation or suggestion on what is indicated within the table.

One method of reading a numeric table is to firstly examine the table title, and column and row headings to understand the context of the data included. Having developed an idea of its purpose and elements, look at the table as a whole and consider the question 'what can we say from this table?'. Answer this by comparing and contrasting the responses indicated by one row or column in relation to another. Are they the same or different? Are they in the proportions (percentages) that you would have expected? What might explain why the proportions are in the pattern found? What conclusions might we draw from this picture? Compare your thoughts to the interpretation suggested by the author. Look at Table 4 and consider what it may reveal about its subject before looking at the next paragraph, which offers a suggestion.

A possible interpretation of the table is that it reveals a gender difference in levels of exercise, where men appear to demonstrate higher levels of exercise than women. Are there reasons that might explain this pattern? Do not forget that this is also a 'self-report' method and we may be unable to confirm this outcome if it is the result of questionnaires (are there any possible differences in the degree of accuracy in this kind of figure provided by males and females?). In addition, a 'p' value would be needed to indicate if this difference in the actual numbers, as opposed to the percentages, is large enough to be more than simply a chance difference.

Table (continued)

Table 4   Those taking more than 30 minutes exercise a week by gender (*n* = 782).

Gender	More than 30 minutes exercise per week	
	Yes (%)	No (%)
Male	246 (62)	154 (38)
Female	168 (44)	214 (56)
Total	414 (53)	368 (47)

How many people were in this fictional study? If you look at the title, the '*n*=' indicates how many people are represented in this table as '*n*' stands for 'number'. If you work out the total for each gender by reading across the rows, you will see that males *n* = 400 and females *n* − 382. The numbers in each group do not have to be exactly the same but it makes comparisons of just the plain or 'raw' numbers sometimes misleading. That is why comparisons between percentages are more useful as both genders are comparable as they are expressed out of a hundred (percent).

Although the table follows the 2×2 format, an extra row has been included showing the column totals, it is still essentially a 2×2 table as a 'totals' row does not indicate a further variable.

The use of tables demonstrates how the researcher can make data and the patterns they contain clearer to the reader; in return, the obligation of the reader is to spend time on the tables and look for the story they reveal.

Note that tables are numbered and titled above what follows, as tables are read from the top down. In contrast, bar groups and histograms have the figure number and title below the figure, as figures are usually read from the bottom up.

See also: Data presentation, quantitative research, critiquing, *p* values.

Thick data (See: Credibility and fieldwork)

Transferability (See: Fittingness)

Triangulation (See: Confirmability and qualitative research designs)

Trustworthiness (See: Credibility)

Type I, Type II, Type III errors

Related to: Inferential statistics, null hypothesis, experimental research.

Definition: An error made by the researcher in relation to the interpretation of the results of an experimental design. This happens when the null hypothesis (which states that there is no difference between the results of the experimental and control group) is either incorrectly rejected, and the data accepted as indicating a difference between the two (*Type I error*), or incorrectly accepting the null hypothesis that there is no difference between the two groups when in fact there is a real difference between them (*Type II error*).

More recently, a *Type III error* has been created to describe a study that asks the wrong question, given the purpose or issue that has prompted the study. This produces an answer or solution that really does not add to our knowledge of the issue.

Application: Research is not an easy activity to carry out nor is it easy to get every aspect of it right. There are two areas highlighted here: firstly, the fundamental importance of getting the research question wording right, given the context of the problem or issue it addresses. This is described as a Type III error, as this idea was developed some time after the development of Type I and Type II errors.

Type I and Type II errors relate to experimental designs where clinical interventions are compared between the experimental and control groups. Randomised controlled trials help the researcher answers the question: 'did the intervention work?' In the planning stage, the traditional scientific approach is to write a null hypothesis to guide the study. This is a statement that suggests that there will be no difference found between the outcome measures of the two groups. This is written hoping that the null hypothesis will be rejected, as a difference between the groups will indicate the success of the intervention.

Once the data are collected, the researcher uses a statistical test of significance to make the decision, should the null hypothesis be accepted and conclude that there is no difference between the groups, or reject the null hypothesis and conclude, they are different and one intervention is more effective than the other. This decision is influenced by the '*p* value' that indicates the probability of a real statistical difference between the results of the two groups. As every study encounters problems, errors do occur, which include the researcher's inability to control everything that might influence the dependent variable, getting a large enough sample and the inaccuracy of data collection tools.

Key revision points: Studies that contain a null hypothesis are susceptible to two major types of error, namely,

- rejecting the null hypothesis when it is true (Type I error);
- accepting the null hypothesis when it is false (Type II error).

Clearly, either of these produces inaccurate conclusions that could be dangerous, or at least result in ineffective knowledge or care. The problem is that such errors are not always apparent, and it is difficult for the reader of a study to know whether either of these errors has taken place. Each error has different influences that should have been considered at the planning and analysis stages. The main influences for both types of errors and some possible actions are summarised in Table 5.

The table demonstrates that experimental studies can lead to errors in the researcher's interpretation of the results. These can be reduced by taking some of the precautions suggested in the table; however, some unknown inaccuracies may still exist.

Type I, Type II, Type III errors (continued)

Table 5   Common problems leading to Type I and Type II errors and possible corrective actions.

Influences	Possible action
Poor choice in level of '*p* value' to decide if there is a clear difference between the two groups	Raising or lowering the *p* value level at which a real difference will be accepted, usually set at $p < 0.05$ or $p < 0.01$, reduces the chance of one of the types of error, but will raise it for the other. The researcher has to decide on which error should be given highest priority to avoid
Data collection tool is not sensitive to all changes in the dependent variable	Use a sensitive tool with high levels of reliability and validity to increase accuracy, or carefully pilot the data collection tool. Accuracy for some tools may be improved with greater training in their use by data collectors
Other unknown or uncontrolled variables influence the outcome measures in the groups	Higher levels of control over data collection and greater examination of the literature to reveal other known influences on the outcome measure
Sample too small to demonstrate statistical changes between groups	Use of 'power calculations' to increase the sample size so that it is large enough for statistical analysis to be sensitive. It is useful to make the sample larger than the target size to compensate for those dropping out of the study

Research is a complex activity, and Type I and Type II errors are a reminder of the need for careful planning of experimental designs and the need to be aware of their limitations. Type III errors also demonstrate the need to get the research question right if we are to develop appropriate knowledge and understanding, and to make best use of research opportunities.

See also: Experimental research, inferential statistics, power analysis.

Unstructured interviews

Related to: Qualitative research, research design, interviews.

Definition: Type of free-flowing 'conversational' interview where the interviewer focusses what may be important to the interviewee and encourages them to raise issues expressed in their own words. In this type of interview, the researcher does not work with a rigid list of questions that are asked in the same way to all respondents, but rather follows the individual's comments and concentrates more on asking for elaborations, clarifications and examples where required.

Application: Interviews are one of best methods of obtaining rich, in-depth information from individuals. Where little is known about a topic, or where the researcher applies the principles of qualitative research, unstructured interviews are the most useful approach to avoid both missing important data and to capture the respondent's viewpoint and agenda.

Key revision points: The goal of interviews is to collect accurate, complete data that avoid bias and achieve the study aim. In qualitative interviews, this is accomplished by ensuring that the interviewer prioritises the thoughts and ideas of the person interviewed, rather than impose the researcher's own thoughts or understanding. This requires a high degree of skill to ensure that information is relevant to the topic but still 'owned' by the interviewee. The interviewer must be continually considering if more depth is required, and further questioning should be pursued, such as 'can you tell me more about x?'.

Unstructured interviews have consequences for data analysis, as it leads to a large amount of words that have to be processed by the researcher. This practical problem is one of the reasons why the analysis of qualitative data is carried out in parallel with data collection. It allows the researcher to identify new relevant themes or issues that may require further investigation in subsequent interviews. It also allows the researcher to identify when the study can be safely stopped as saturation has been reached and no new themes are emerging.

See also: Qualitative research, interviews, research design, open questions.

Rapid Research Methods for Nurses, Midwives and Health Professionals,
First Edition. Colin Rees.
© 2016 John Wiley & Sons, Ltd. Published 2016 by John Wiley & Sons, Ltd.

Unstructured observations

Related to: Qualitative research, research design, observation.

Definition: A method of collecting observational data that takes into account the total setting and events rather than a structured checklist of items or aspects covering a narrow view.

Application: This method of observation relates to qualitative studies such as ethnographic research, where the researcher sets out to record and understand events as they unfold, in order to get a total picture of a situation.

Such studies have the advantage of depth and 'reality' by providing a clear account of processes and systems that may be unconscious actions to those pursuing them. Such actions may be 'invisible' and out of the reach of respondents if they were asked to recount them in a questionnaire or interview.

Key revision points: Unstructured observation, where the researcher collects in-depth and prolonged observational data, is ideal for qualitative research that seeks to uncover valuable accounts of situations and events.

It does require a complex of skills from the observer in being able to record information in a sustained way. Observers can suffer from 'observational drift' where the researcher's thoughts and fatigue reduce the accuracy of the data. The role of the observer in terms of the awareness of those being observed has also to be considered. Although options range from 'covert', where the act of observing is hidden from those in the study, to 'overt observation', where it is clear that observation is being carried out. However, as there are ethical issues of informed consent, confidentially and possible harm involved in covert observations, particularly where it takes place on health premises, ethics committees are reluctant to support it.

Unstructured observation studies produce huge amounts of descriptive data that require careful categorisation and interpretation, making it a complex form of research. However, the rewards of this type of study are immense.

See also: Observation, research methods, ethical issues, qualitative approaches, ethnographic research.

Validity

Related to: Critical evaluation, data analysis.

Definition: The extent to which a data gathering tool can be demonstrated to measure the concept of interest to the researcher.

Application: Within healthcare, researchers attempt to gain a better understanding of complex and abstract concepts, such as resilience, quality of life and trust. The problem for the quantitative researcher is to use a tool or scale that is capable of accurately measuring these concepts. This is the issue covered by the concept of validity, which along with reliability, bias and rigour is used to evaluate the quality of research studies as part of critical analysis.

Key revision points: When critically analysing published research studies, the methods section should indicate the confidence the researcher had in the tools they used to collect the data. Some methods section may have a subheading 'validity and reliability'; if this appears, the reliability aspect will focus on the accuracy and consistency of the measurements, whereas the validity aspect will outline how the researcher developed questions or scales used to measure the key concepts and their certainty that the tools did measure those concepts. This is not an easy task for the researcher and the use of the same or similar tools by previous researchers is often used to argue that validity has been achieved.

Face validity: This is sometimes mentioned as a way of checking whether experts agree that 'on the face of it', the questions included in data collection are relevant and judge a fundamental component of the concept being measured.

In randomised controlled trials, there are a number of 'threats to validity' that can seriously limit the accuracy of the interpretation of the results. These include firstly elements related to *internal validity*, that is, those aspects within a particular trial that might negatively influence the interpretations of the results. Internal validity examines whether the intervention has produced a change in the dependent variable (outcome) and alternative explanations have been considered.

Internal threats to validity include the following:

- History: changes in society or the local community outside the study happening at the same time as the study that may have produced the outcome rather than the independent variable.

- Maturity: changes due to developments in the individual such as physical maturity or gaining insights or understandings that were not a result of the independent variable. Maturity can be applied to short time period as it relates simply to changes due to changes over time.

Rapid Research Methods for Nurses, Midwives and Health Professionals,
First Edition. Colin Rees.
© 2016 John Wiley & Sons, Ltd. Published 2016 by John Wiley & Sons, Ltd.

Validity (continued)

- Attrition (also called mortality but does not necessarily mean some of the sample died): difficulties in comparing the experimental and control group results as a result of some people dropping out of one group causing an imbalance in important characteristics between the groups. Although the two groups may have been comparable at the beginning of the study, once their composition has changed, it is no longer possible to be sure that the intervention is the only factor that could be responsible for post-test differences.

- Testing: changes in post-test differences, especially in knowledge or attitude, due to respondents remembering the pre-test questions and responses, or respondents changing due to reflecting on issues raised by the pre-test and not the consequence of any intervention.

- Instrumentation: change influenced by alterations in the accuracy of the instrument at the post-test stage.

Similarly, there can be threats to *external validity* where interpretations of the results are influenced by limitations in being able to transfer the results from one particular study site or sample to other locations. These can include the following:

- Reactivity: changes due to people behaving differently because they are part of a study and feel different (sometimes referred to as the *Hawthorne effect*);

- Novelty: changes due to the impact of new or unusual features of the intervention that stimulate change rather than any changes in the therapeutic effect;

- Sample selection: the difficulty in arguing that those who elect to take part in a study, particularly a complex or long duration study, are typical of the larger population. The threat is one of bias and unrepresentativeness of the sample that limits the findings to the study group and reduces the generalisability of the results. There may also be problems in applying the findings from one country to another due to subtle or not so subtle differences between them that make application of the results difficult.

All of these issues demonstrate that claiming a study demonstrates a cause-and-effect relationship between an intervention and an outcome measure is not straightforward. Although randomisation and blinding/masking are ways of overcoming some of these problems, it may not be possible to deal with all the problems involved in claiming validity in a study.

See also: Critique, bias, Hawthorne effect, reliability, rigour, experimental research, confounding variable.

Variable

Related to: Research process.

Definition: The basic building block of research that names the aspect(s) in a study that varies or changes, and about which the researcher gathers data. Depending on the research approach, there can be one, two or more variables in a study.

Application: The variable is probably one of the most important elements in any study; without one, there is no study. In experimental studies, it is the element the researcher attempts to change or modify and is controlled and measured in the study. What gives a variable form and a reality within research is a *concept definition* and *operational definition*.

Concept definitions are similar to dictionary definitions in that they explain or outline what is meant by the word used to describe the variable. This enables everyone to share a clear and similar understanding of what is being examined.

In quantitative research, the operational definition details the way in which the concept is measured and therefore 'operationalised'. This can take the form of a measuring instrument such as a thermometer, weighing scales, or attitude or other scale, such as a depression or anxiety scale.

Key revision points: In critically examining a research study, one of the preliminary stages is to identify the variables concerned. These may be identified in the title, but will usually appear in the aim, as that indicates the focus of data collection. Well-written studies will give a clear concept and operational definition for the major variables early in the study. In experimental studies, there will be a dependent variable, which is the outcome variable such as level of pain or anxiety, and an independent variable that forms the intervention introduced by the researcher, such as a form of motivation, exercise system or pain-reducing regime. The need for a clear definition and a way of measuring each variable with a reliable tool can clearly be seen from this.

In qualitative research, there will be a variable that forms the focus of the study but may be thought of more as an issue or a behavioural or experiential concept such as resilience or hope. Although there may be attempts to define these with a concept definition, there will not be an operational definition as qualitative research is not concerned with measuring anything and does not use a scale or other form of tool that produces numeric results.

Concept and operational definitions are also important when it comes to reviews of the literature. They enable the author to ensure that studies can be combined or examined together by ensuring that the concept and operational definitions of variables are compatible. Differences in the definitions would explain why the results for some studies are dissimilar or at odds with each other as they would be looking at slightly different variables and measuring them in different ways that make comparisons or amalgamation difficult or unhelpful.

See also: Dependent variable, independent variable, concept definition, operational definition.